Penguin Books
Hypnotherapy for Everyon

Dr Ruth Lever qualified fror
with the degrees of M.B., B.S.
has included work in paediatrics, psychiatry and public health
and she has an M.Sc. in social medicine from London University.

For four and a half years she was Medical Officer in Charge of
Troops at a large Army depot and it was during this period that
she started to study and practise various alternative therapies
including acupuncture, hypnosis, healing and nutrition counselling. Since leaving Army practice, she has started writing on
various aspects of orthodox and alternative medicine and is the
author of *Acupuncture for Everyone* (Penguin, 1987). She has
appeared regularly on the TVS programme *Problem Page* and
writes a weekly column in *Best* magazine.

She is now in practice with her husband, who is a homoeo-
path.

RUTH LEVER

HYPNOTHERAPY FOR EVERYONE

PENGUIN BOOKS

PENGUIN BOOKS

Published by the Penguin Group
27 Wrights Lane, London W8 5TZ, England
Viking Penguin Inc., 40 West 23rd Street, New York, New York 10010, USA
Penguin Books Australia Ltd, Ringwood, Victoria, Australia
Penguin Books Canada Ltd, 2801 John Street, Markham, Ontario, Canada L3R 1B4
Penguin Books (NZ) Ltd, 182–190 Wairau Road, Auckland 10, New Zealand

Penguin Books Ltd, Registered Offices: Harmondsworth, Middlesex, England

First published 1988

Made and printed in Great Britain by
Richard Clay Ltd, Bungay, Suffolk
Filmset in 11/13 Monophoto Plantin

For my parents, Hetty and Lionel Lever,
with love and gratitude

CONTENTS

ACKNOWLEDGEMENTS

My sincere thanks to the many hypnotherapists whose lectures and writings have inspired my study of hypnosis in all its aspects.

And a huge thank you to my husband who took time to sit and read through the drafts of this book, and who offered invaluable advice.

Note

Throughout most of this book, 'he' is used in general references to doctors, hypnotherapists and patients, although in passages dealing with conditions that affect women more often than men, the patient is referred to as 'she'. The intention of the author – herself a woman – is, naturally, not to ignore the existence of women in all three categories, but to avoid the irritating repetition of 'he or she'.

CHAPTER ONE

WHAT IS

HYPNOSIS?

Of all the complementary therapies, hypnosis is probably the one about which people have the most preconceived ideas and misconceptions. In many cases, a patient's first contact with a particular therapy (homoeopathy or acupuncture, for example) is when he goes to a therapist for treatment. He may have read somewhere that 'arthritis responds well to acupuncture' or someone may have told him that 'homoeopathy worked wonders for my sinusitis' but, very often, all he knows about the system that he is going to try is that it doesn't use drugs. Therefore he is able to go for treatment with an open mind.

With hypnosis, however, the picture is rather different. Most people are unaware that it can be used to treat a large number of conditions, although many know that it is a useful aid for those who are trying to give up smoking. But almost everyone has, at one time or another, seen a stage hypnotist or has read a book or seen a film in which people are hypnotized and made to do whatever the hypnotist desires. They have, therefore, a rather terrifying – and quite inaccurate – view of hypnosis. What they have seen or read has made it seem that the mind of the subject is completely in the control of the hypnotist and that, as a result, the subject can be made to do things against his will. The use of hypnosis in helping patients to give up smoking reinforces this idea, since the impression is given that they are *made* to stop. Even those patients who have been advised by their general practitioners to try some hypnotherapy, or those who actually know people who have benefited from such treatment, often go to their first appointment in a spirit of trepidation. It is important, therefore, to discuss these misconceptions from the word go, and to show where they are incorrect. Going to see a practitioner of whose therapy you understand very little is difficult enough; going to see someone who practises a therapy which seems both obscure and threatening is probably enough to make many people decide that they'd rather not try it in the first place.

Perhaps the misconception it is most important to dispel is that which says that hypnosis works by allowing the hypnotist to take control of the mind of the subject. If this really were the case, one could envisage all sorts of terrible things happening if one were unfortunate enough to get into the hands of an unscrupulous hypnotist. One might be made to do all sorts of things, perhaps even commit crimes, against one's will, or one might be made to divulge secrets that one would rather keep hidden. Fortunately, such anxieties are groundless, since hypnosis cannot make one do anything to which one would normally object. This, of course, is why hypnosis doesn't always work for people who are trying to give up smoking. Some people really enjoy smoking and are only trying to give up because pressure is being put on them by husbands, wives, parents or general practitioners; or they may feel that they ought to give up, for financial or health reasons, without really wanting to give up. For these people, hypnotherapy will be of no use at all. If, however, the patient is strongly motivated to give up, then hypnosis will reinforce his own determination and, in this way, will make his transition from smoker to non-smoker a great deal easier than it might otherwise have been.

People often ask why it is that stage hypnotists can make their subjects do foolish things under hypnosis if it is true that they do not have control over them. The answer to this is quite simple, although one needs to look at the whole of the hypnotist's act to realize how it works. He will usually start by asking everyone in the audience to do a few tests, so that he can see who is likely to be a good hypnotic subject. These tests are often introduced as a sort of game that everyone participates in, so that the audience does not realize that it is being tested. By the end of the tests, most of the audience will be in a 'party mood' and ready to join in the show. Then the hypnotist will pick out a number of people who look to him as though they are likely to be good subjects and he will ask them to come up on stage. Anyone who doesn't want to be a part of the entertainment is likely to refuse, at this point, to join in. So the hypnotist can be fairly sure that those people who do come up will be willing to play along and that, as long as he doesn't ask them to do anything completely against their principles (like taking their clothes off) they will go along with him. He then tries out various tests on them and, out of those 15 or 20 whom he initially selected, he picks perhaps four or five who seem to him not only to be good subjects but also good sports.

A few years before I became interested in hypnotherapy, I was invited to 'come up on stage' by a hypnotist and was chosen as one of his final four subjects. We were asked to do all manner of silly things which I knew perfectly well were silly at the time – but I went along with it because it was a bit of fun and I didn't want to spoil the man's act. This is not to say that stage hypnosis is always safe. It is certainly possible for subjects to become upset or embarrassed when they find themselves doing silly things. But any suggestion which the subject finds truly objectionable will be ignored.

However, hypnotism, as it is used by stage hypnotists, really has very little in common with hypnotherapy other than the basic technique. It is important to remember that the sole aim of the stage hypnotist is to entertain and, to that end, he may make hypnosis look quite different from what it actually is. Because his subjects have willingly gone up on stage, it is unlikely that they will resist hypnosis. But it is perfectly possible to refuse to go into a trance – indeed it is impossible to hypnotize someone unless he really wants to be hypnotized. (Paradoxically, if someone is overkeen to be hypnotized, he may find that he does not go into trance. It's like willing yourself to go to sleep – it just doesn't work.) However, patients who have had their initial fears dispelled about the process of hypnosis are usually fairly relaxed about the induction and go under quite easily. And the more often they are hypnotized, the easier it gets, since they become more and more confident about the technique and its benefits. But it is, of course, important that, from the first session, the patient knows that it is he who is in control and not the therapist.

Because the patient is in control, he cannot be made to stay in hypnosis if he should decide that he wants to wake up. Usually patients enjoy being in hypnosis and have no wish to cut the session short, but occasionally someone will bring himself out of trance and it is not uncommon, after the first session, for a patient to say, 'I felt that I could wake up at any time.' (If one asks why he didn't do so, the answer is usually, 'Oh, I didn't *want* to – I just felt that I *could*.') However, there are occasions on which a patient wishes to wake. He may wake automatically if a suggestion is made that is so contrary to his own ideas that he finds it offensive or alarming. This is, therefore, an additional safeguard against being made to do anything against one's will. But there may be other reasons why the patient wakes. For example, there was a woman who had an appointment at an afternoon clinic which was running about 20 minutes late. Halfway through her session, she suddenly woke herself up, saying, 'I'm terribly sorry, but I've got to go and pick the children up from school.' So, even though she was in a moderately deep trance, she was aware of the time and of what she had to do and was able to wake herself up in order to do it.

We always talk about waking up from hypnosis and about hypnotic sleep, so it is quite natural that people who have not been hypnotized should imagine that being in a trance is rather like being asleep. Indeed, the word 'hypnosis' is derived from the Greek *hypnos*, which means sleep. The word itself, therefore, can make the patient apprehensive: having things 'done to you' while you are asleep is reminiscent of having an operation – something that most people are, understandably, quite nervous about. But, in fact, the word is misleading, since the hypnotized patient is far from being oblivious to everything as though he were asleep but, on the contrary, is able to hear and respond to everything the therapist says to him.

However, the patient's reaction to his surroundings may vary according to the depth of trance he has reached. Suppose a patient has come to his appointment with his wife. If he sits with his eyes shut while the therapist talks to his wife about him, at some stage he may well open his eyes and join in the conversation. If, however, the patient has already been put into a light trance, he will listen to the conversation between his wife and the therapist but will probably have no great desire to join in. If he has gone into a fairly deep trance, he will hear what the other two are saying but he will not actively listen. However, at no time, no matter how deep the trance, is the patient 'unconscious'. The way in which patients become distanced from their surroundings while in a trance was nicely demonstrated by a woman who was being treated by a doctor shortly after he had first started to use hypnosis. She was already in a trance when the telephone on his desk started to ring. It was quickly answered on the extension but he was concerned that it might have disturbed her. When he woke her up, he asked her about this and she said, 'Oh no, it didn't disturb me at all – but I was aware that it had disturbed you!'

Hypnosis, therefore, is not a form of unconsciousness but, rather, an altered form of consciousness in which the patient is more open to suggestion than he normally would be and in which a corridor is opened between the conscious and the subconscious mind. It is the subconscious mind that is responsible for our automatic reactions and therefore for our response to stress (causing migraines, rashes, asthma and so on). It also bottles up memories of things that have happened to us in the past and acts automatically upon those memories. In this way, phobias may develop. Opening up a corridor to the subconscious mind may allow it to accept suggestions which it can use to promote automatic reactions that will benefit the patient, and may allow old 'redundant' memories to be recognized as no longer important.

Let us suppose that someone has gone to see a hypnotherapist in order to give up smoking. The therapist puts him into a hypnotic trance and gives him certain suggestions, perhaps telling him that cigarettes will taste dreadful in future and that he will have no desire to smoke. Now, if the patient was in a state similar to sleep, the therapist's words would be lost on him, for he would not hear them and they would have no effect. In hypnosis, however, he is fully aware of what the therapist is saying. The trance has the effect of temporarily removing the critical faculty of the brain – in other words, the mind accepts the suggestion that this will happen, without wondering why on earth it should. Therefore the patient will believe what he is told about the evil-tasting cigarettes and his lack of desire to smoke, although, had he been told such things when he was awake, he might well have dismissed them as nonsense. Oddly enough, even if the hypnotized patient feels uncertain about the efficacy of the suggestion, it may still work.

An example of this was a patient who was inclined to develop a migraine as soon as she became upset about anything. Unfortunately, she was going through a period when she had a lot of problems and she was getting upset frequently, with a resulting increase in the number of her migraines. She was told, while she was in hypnosis, that she would be able to cope with her problems and would be able to remain calm, not allowing things to upset her, and therefore her migraine would not develop. When she woke up, however, she confessed that, while the therapist had been saying these reassuring things, her mind had been retorting, 'That's what you think!' In view of this, her chances of getting better seemed small. However, when she went to her next appointment, she reported that not only was she coping better and staying calmer but she was having fewer migraines.

Although this patient was able to 'answer back' with her conscious mind, her subconscious obviously had accepted the suggestions given to her by the therapist, since they were in her own best interests. However, had they not been beneficial, then it, too, would have rejected them. An episode from my own experience illustrates this. When I first became interested in hypnotherapy, I attended a tutorial with some five or six other doctors at which our tutor wanted to demonstrate that one can make the patient forget certain things while in hypnosis. Choosing me as the subject, he hypnotized me and then told me that when he tapped his pen on the table, I would forget my name for 30 seconds. But I knew that I didn't want to forget my name, and my subconscious mind evidently knew that there was no reason to override this conscious decision, so that, when the tutor tapped his pen on the table and asked me what my name was, I told him. 'Ah,' he said, 'she obviously doesn't want to forget her name. Let's choose something less threatening.' So he told me that when he tapped his pen on the table, I would forget where I lived. But, being awkward, I didn't want to forget that, either, so the same thing happened – he tapped his pen on the table and asked me my address, and I told him.

It will be clear from what I have said of my own experience and of patients' comments after coming out of hypnosis that it is quite usual for the subject to recall what has happened while he has been in a trance. The idea that one forgets everything that has occurred as soon as one wakes is yet another popular myth – and quite an alarming one. This is the stuff that novels are made of – the hero (or heroine) is hypnotized and only you, the reader, know what instructions he has been given, since he awakes unable to remember anything that has been said. But this is fiction. In fact, it is quite rare for a patient spontaneously to forget what has happened during a session of hypnosis. Those that do will have been in a very deep trance, and such deep levels are uncommon. The reason for this is that only a certain proportion of subjects are capable of going very deep and only a few of these will do so without a great deal of work on the part of the hypnotist. Since a very deep trance is quite unnecessary for most types of treatment, it usually only occurs in the very few patients who are naturally deep subjects. Thus the vast majority will go only into a light or medium depth of trance, from which they will emerge remembering everything.

Occasionally it can be beneficial to the treatment for the patient to forget one or more things that have come up during hypnosis. But, as I proved when I refused to forget my name and address, he will only forget those things which he is happy to forget. The suggestion that certain facts will be forgotten may be given when a patient has been recalling disturbing incidents in his past with which his conscious mind is not yet ready to deal. For example, a patient may have developed a phobia as the result of a frightening incident that occurred when he was a child. He may then have blotted out the incident from his conscious mind but kept the fear associated with it, which has now turned into a phobia. In the treatment of his condition it may be important for its cause to be brought to the fore while he is in hypnosis, but the memory may still be more than his mind can deal with. Therefore, the form of suggestion that is often used is, 'You will forget anything that you have remembered during this session with which your conscious mind is not yet ready to deal. However, when your conscious mind can cope with them, these memories will slowly come back to you.' Thus it is the patient's own mind that decides what he is ready to remember, and when.

It can be seen that it is much easier to describe hypnosis in terms of what it is not than in terms of what it is. This may be the reason why it has never been called by any name that really describes what it is or does. 'Hypnosis', as I have said, is misleading, since it implies sleep. Previous names are equally vague. The trance state has been known for thousands of years but in the seventeenth and eighteenth centuries it became known as 'animal magnetism' in the mistaken belief that it had something to do with the flow of magnetic forces through the subject. The greatest exponent of animal magnetism in the eighteenth century was Dr Anton Mesmer. In the following century, especially as the magnetic theory became discredited, the term 'animal magnetism' was replaced by 'mesmerism'. This is still used, particularly in the sense of 'I was quite mesmerized by it', meaning 'I was enthralled'. The term 'hypnosis' was only coined in the mid-nineteenth century and is just a recent name for a very ancient technique.

CHAPTER TWO

A SHORT HISTORY

OF HYPNOSIS

Although Mesmer was the first to use hypnosis on a grand scale in the treatment of disease, his practice was based on a theory that was first proposed in the seventeenth century by a German named Athanasius Kirchir. Kirchir maintained that disease occurred when a magnetic fluid which ran through the body became disturbed. This theory was followed up a hundred years or so later by Father Maximilian Hell, a Jesuit priest. He was also the official astronomer to the Austrian court and it is probable that it was as a scientist rather than as a cleric that he first became interested in magnetism. He started to treat patients by strapping magnetized iron plates to the diseased areas of their bodies, on the premise that if the magnetic fluid was disturbed, it should be possible to restore it to normality by bringing it into contact with a normal magnetic field. Mesmer was a friend of Father Hell (they were probably brought together by a mutual interest in astronomy, a subject Mesmer had studied at university) and it was through him that he started to use magnets in the treatment of his own patients. Popular imagination sees Mesmer as a quack in fancy clothes, tricking gullible people by using techniques of which he knew very little. However, he was a qualified physician and, before his experiments with animal magnetism, well respected.

Mesmer came from a poor family but was an able student and won a scholarship to the Jesuit university of Dillingen in Bavaria. There he studied logic, metaphysics, theology,

Latin, Greek, public speaking, philosophy and science. However, he had no vocation for the priesthood (it is probable that he chose the Jesuit university simply because the scholarship was offered). So, at the end of his four years of studies, he moved to the larger Bavarian university of Ingoldstadt. It seems that initially he intended to pursue a similar course, since he enrolled in the faculty of theology, but he soon changed his mind and abandoned the study of religion in favour of physics, mathematics, astronomy and languages. He evidently had a voracious appetite for learning and, when he reached the end of his four-year course at Ingoldstadt, he enrolled at the University of Vienna to study law. However, by the end of his first year at Vienna he had found his true vocation and had transferred to the faculty of medicine. He finally qualified as a doctor, aged 32, in 1766. This was a time when many new and wonderful discoveries were being made in the world of science and, for someone with Mesmer's breadth of knowledge and enquiring mind, it must have been tempting to try to link up all the new data – physical, chemical and biological. He was very influenced by the work of Isaac Newton on gravity and felt that this newly discovered force must have some effect on the human body. This seemed to tie in with the idea of magnetic forces being implicated in disease and, in a paper which he wrote in 1776, entitled 'The Influence of the Planets on the Human Body', he proposed that the absence of disease was dependent upon a balance being maintained between the magnetic fluid in the patient's body and that in the external universe.

Not long after he qualified, Mesmer married Maria Anna von Posch, who was a wealthy widow from an aristocratic family and some ten years his senior. Thanks to her, he was able to establish himself in polite society in Vienna and to set up his medical practice among the well-to-do residents of the city. And it was on a friend, or possibly relative, of

hers that Mesmer first experimented with 'animal magnetism'. Maria Anna had invited this young woman, Franzl
(Francisca) Oesterlin to live with them. She was in her late
twenties and had suffered, over a period of two years, from
a whole catalogue of ailments such as vomiting, toothache,
earache, depression and fainting fits. Since she was living
in his house, it was natural that she should become one of
Mesmer's patients (maybe it was with a view to getting her
treated that Maria Anna installed her in the house in the
first place). At first he used orthodox methods but found
that, although she seemed to recover, she would then relapse again. It seemed to him that the ebb and flow of
illness in Franzl was like the action of a magnetic force and
he therefore decided to treat her with the magnetic therapy
of which he had read and heard. His friend Father Hell
acquired the magnets for him and Franzl was treated – and
cured. Flushed with success, Mesmer tried the therapy on
other patients suffering from complaints such as hysteria,
depression and fits, with encouraging results. In the following year (1775) he treated Wilhelm Bauer, Professor of
Mathematics at Vienna University, and cured him of
sleepwalking.

If Mesmer had been a poor country doctor, experi-
menting on the peasantry with a seemingly outlandish
treatment, it is probable that he would have been left alone
to continue his practice as he saw fit, perhaps being labelled
a harmless eccentric. But he was not in a position where
this could happen. On the contrary, he was a well-known
figure in Vienna and among his patients were members of
the aristocracy and the intelligentsia as well as the wealthy.
People began to talk about his methods and his apparent
cures, and other doctors started to form their own opinions
about what he was doing. Some, more open-minded than
the rest, tried the magnetic treatment for themselves. Of
these, some found it helpful and continued to use it, while

others, whose patients did not get better, discarded it. The less open-minded condemned it out of hand as quackery. However, Mesmer was anxious that the medical profession should recognize his treatment as useful, if, perhaps, unorthodox. He therefore sent a report of his work to the Berlin Academy of Sciences, where it was studied by members of the mathematics and physics department. They chose to ignore Mesmer's hypothesis that the magnetic force involved was one which could be communicated from one person to another and that the magnets simply acted as a channel for this, and reported that, although they thought that magnetic force might have some influence on the human body, they doubted whether the magnets themselves were effective in producing the cures that were claimed.

Of course, the practice of strapping magnets to a patient's body is nothing like the practice of hypnosis as we know it and, at first glance, there would seem to be no apparent connection between 'animal magnetism' and hypnotherapy. But Mesmer's ideas about a magnetic force being communicated from therapist to patient suggest that, from the first, he was doing more than just applying magnets. It seems likely that he was putting many, if not all, of his patients into a hypnotic trance and he must certainly have been successful in a good percentage of his treatments, for it is unlikely that patients would have continued to attend his clinics if the therapy was of no use. One might, of course, theorize that Mesmer was using something other than hypnosis. If a healer who works by 'laying on hands' were to read about Mesmer's work, he might equate it with his own. Many healers agree that most doctors can heal with their hands and that it is probably this innate ability that led them to study medicine in the first place. So, taking this theory a stage further, it is possible that Mesmer, while believing that he was communicating a magnetic force to the patient through his hands and through the magnets, was, in fact, using the 'healing force' used by healers. However, even if he was a healer – which is pure supposition – this cannot have been the whole story. The ability to heal is a very individual thing, being very strong in some people, weaker or non-existent in others. But the ability to hypnotize is something that can be learned by anyone. Later in his life, Mesmer taught a large number of people to perform his therapy successfully and even taught a Swiss surgeon to treat himself by sending him instructions in a letter. This would be quite possible with hypnosis but very unlikely to happen with healing alone.

From the first, Mesmer was aware that his treatment worked best in conditions which were produced or controlled by the patient's mind. In some cases, such as that of a Hungarian baron who suffered from severe spasms in his neck, he did not even use magnets but simply talked to the patient, in the way that a hypnotherapist might today.

When Mesmer was invited by the Munich Academy of Sciences to demonstrate his methods to its members, it seemed that he was starting to get the official recognition that he craved. The Academy, unlike that of Berlin, was impressed by the demonstration and offered Mesmer membership. Interestingly enough, in view of the theory I have just put forward that Mesmer might have been a healer, the Academy also asked his opinion on a certain Father Gassner who had been curing people by the laying on of hands. Mesmer's answer was that Father Gassner was, without realizing it, curing his patients by the use of animal magnetism.

All went well until Mesmer was asked to treat Maria-Theresa von Paradies, the 18-year-old daughter of the Emperor's private secretary. Although she had been blind from the age of four, Maria-Theresa was a talented pianist and, thanks to a pension granted to her by the Empress, had been able to study with the best teachers. It seems that Dr Stoerk, the chief court physician, was aware that her blindness was a hysterical complaint, not a physical one, and had treated her for several years with a variety of barbaric therapies which were then in use for psychiatric problems, including leeches, purgatives and electric shocks to her eyes. Finally, she had been pronounced incurable by a top eye specialist. But then Mesmer took a hand in her treatment and within a month her sight started to return.

Dr Stoerk was courteous enough to acknowledge Mesmer's success but other physicians were outraged that Mesmer could cure (or claim to cure), using bizarre methods, a condition for which they could do nothing. Reports started to circulate that the girl was really still blind. Her father, informed that her pension might be withdrawn if she regained her sight, demanded that the treatment be stopped. As a result of all the tension, the improvement in Maria-Theresa's condition could not be maintained and her blindness returned. Her father then had a change of heart and asked Mesmer to continue to treat her, which he did. It seems that she was one of the patients for whom he did not use magnets, being able to 'magnetize' (or hypnotize) her without them. After another four weeks of treatment, her sight was, once more, returning. But her father, probably under pressure from those who were hostile to Mesmer, would not allow her to admit that she could see, making her behave as though she was still blind and telling people that she had not been cured. In addition to all the stress that she was being put under by the politics of her treatment, poor Maria-Theresa found that, with her sight restored, her skill at the piano was diminished and, finally, she relapsed again into blindness. This, of course, gave added weight to the argument of the Viennese physicians that Mesmer was nothing but a charlatan and, as a result, the University of Vienna stated

publicly that his treatment was worthless. With this con-
demnation, Mesmer felt that he could no longer continue
to practise in his own country and he left for France.

In May 1778, Mesmer set up a clinic a few miles outside
Paris and was fortunate enough to attract the interest of Dr
Charles d'Eslon, who was to become a loyal patron and
supporter of his work. D'Eslon was a person of some
standing in the world of French medicine, being the personal physician of the Comte d'Artois who, later, was to
become King Charles X of France. Once again, Mesmer
became established in the upper echelons of society and
patients flocked to see him. Indeed, he had so many re-
quests for treatment that he had to devise a method of
treating more than one patient at a time. He therefore developed his 'baquet' – a huge oak tub filled with water and
containing iron filings, powdered glass and phials of
'magnetized' water arranged in concentric circles. A lid
covered the tub and through it ran jointed iron rods which
'connected' the patients to the mixture within. Each patient
applied one of the rods to the affected part of his body.
Then, sitting silently round the tub, all the patients joined
hands while Mesmer fixed each in turn with his eyes, waved
his hands around them and touched them with an iron
wand. Around the walls were mirrors which reflected
carefully positioned lights; there were heavy curtains and
thick carpets and, in the background, musicians played
softly. Once more, satisfied patients spread the word about
his treatment and soon he was unable to cope with the
numbers who wished to be seen, even by using the *baquet*.
By this time, he had decided that any object could convey
the vital magnetic fluid and so, attaching cords to the
branches of a large tree, he asked his patients to sit and
hold the cords while he treated them.

But despite his undoubted success with the public,
Mesmer was still hankering after official approval. To try

to achieve this, d'Eslon managed to arrange for three rep-resentatives of the French Faculty of Medicine to attend the clinic to investigate Mesmer's claims. However, al-though they watched patients being treated, they main-tained that they could not comment on the results since they had been unable personally to examine the patients before the therapy began. And, in the end, the investigation was dropped.

In 1780, d'Eslon published a report entitled 'Observa-tions on Animal Magnetism', in which he advocated the use of the therapy. This lost him the good will of the Faculty of Medicine, who accused him of using his prominent posi-tion to promote the activities of a German mountebank – an interesting turn of phrase which suggests that, had Mesmer been French, the Faculty might have felt less hostile towards him. D'Eslon suggested that a study be carried out to compare a group of patients treated by Mesmer with a group treated by orthodox methods. How-ever, the Faculty was not going to be persuaded into open-minded investigation. The suggestion was refused and d'Eslon was told that if he had not rejected Mesmer's theories within a year, he would lose his membership.

The following year, after a further unsuccessful attempt to achieve 'respectability' and a short period spent away from Paris, made necessary by his despondency at its fail-ure, Mesmer set up an organization which he named the 'Society of Harmony'. Into this he accepted people who wished to learn about his treatment and how to use it. There was a great deal of interest and among those who enrolled were noblemen, priests, businessmen and even some doctors. Some of those who took the training were given certificates and allowed to set up their own practices – eventually Mesmer trained about 300 people and some 40 provincial Societies of Harmony were set up.

In 1784 d'Eslon, still pursuing Mesmer's dream of recognition by practitioners of orthodox medicine, managed to persuade the Queen to influence her husband to set up a royal commission. Five members of the French Academy of Science and four from the Faculty of Medicine were chosen and asked to examine the therapeutic value of animal magnetism. The chairman of the commission was Benjamin Franklin, inventor, author, statesman and philanthropist, who at that time was the American ambassador to the French court. The deputy chairman was the astronomer Jean-Sylvain Bailly. Also from the Academy of Science was Antoine Lavoisier, a brilliant chemist, who is remembered for isolating from the air the gas which he named oxygen, and for devising the system of atomic weights. From the Faculty of Medicine came Dr Joseph Guillotin, whose name is remembered in connection with the instrument that was, nine years later, to chop off the king's head.

The members of the commission decided, first of all, to subject themselves to treatment by animal magnetism. But when they did so, they felt nothing and therefore came to the conclusion that magnetism had no effect on healthy patients. So they picked some patients to be used as guinea-pigs. However, these were not patients who would have gone to Mesmer's clinic of their own accord and the more educated among them were sceptical about the therapy. Since hypnosis will not work on hostile subjects, the only patients who responded were those from the 'lower classes'. After due deliberation, the commission came to the conclusion that Mesmer's cures could only be explained if either the cure or the illness was in the mind of the patient. This, of course, is a fairly crude description of the sorts of conditions treatable by hypnosis, which will alleviate symptoms caused by anxiety, tension and other states of mind and which will promote 'mind over matter' to enable patients to overcome pain and other disabilities. However, in the eighteenth century, such a verdict could only mean that Mesmer was a charlatan playing on the susceptibility of gullible patients with vivid imaginations.

The Royal Medical Society of Paris had been somewhat offended that it had not been asked to appoint members to sit on the royal commission and so, at the same time that Benjamin Franklin and his colleagues were deliberating, it set up its own committee of four members to investigate animal magnetism. One of the four produced a minority report in Mesmer's favour but the other three came to the conclusion that not only was his treatment useless but it could also be dangerous. Following the publication of the reports of the two commissions, the University of Paris made it known that any physician under its control who practised animal magnetism would have his licence to practise medicine withdrawn.

This was the end of Mesmer's practice and he returned to Lake Constance, near his birthplace, where he spent nearly 30 years in retirement before dying in 1815 at the age of 81. However, animal magnetism did not die with him. Although he had stopped practising, others continued to use the therapy.

One of these was the Abbé José Custodio di Faria, a Portuguese who, two years before Mesmer's death, gave a series of public demonstrations of animal magnetism in Paris. It seems that he did not meet with the hostility which Mesmer's encountered – possibly because attitudes were different in post-Revolution France or, more likely, because he was not a doctor trying to prove a radical new therapy to other, more conservative, doctors. Like Mesmer, he maintained that the power of animal magnetism lay with both the therapist and the patient and that, for the therapy to be effective, both must work together. This, of course, is still true of hypnosis as it is practised today. However, unlike Mesmer, di Faria dispensed with the 'stage manage-

ment' of heavy curtains and soft music and with the pan-
tomime of waving his hands around. Instead, he just asked
the patients to relax and to feel themselves going to sleep.
This is very similar to the method used by some modern
hypnotherapists.

It was one of Mesmer's pupils, the Marquis Chastenet
de Puysegur, who made the important discovery that some
patients could open their eyes and talk, although still
'magnetized'. In modern hypnotherapy, it is not unusual
for a patient to be asked questions while he is still in a
trance. Not only does this enable the therapist to have a
clearer idea of how the patient is reacting to the treatment
but it also allows him to combine other psychological
therapeutic techniques with the hypnosis. The ability to
open one's eyes while in hypnosis is associated with a particularly deep level of trance and is now known as som-
nambulism.

These pupils of Mesmer, as well as continuing to practise
his therapy, also taught the technique, in modified form, to
others. Perhaps one of the most important of the next
generation of students was an English physician named
John Elliotson. A Londoner and son of a chemist, Elliotson
learned about animal magnetism from Richard Chenevix,
FRS, who had been a pupil of the Abbé di Faria, and from
the Baron Dupotet de Sennevoy, who had been a pupil of
Mesmer's himself. Born in 1791, he went to Edinburgh
University, where he qualified as a doctor, and then continued his studies on the Continent, at Jesus College, Cam-
bridge, and at Guy's and St Thomas's hospitals. He set up
in practice in London and, in 1817, was appointed assistant
physician at St Thomas's hospital. Six years later, he rose to
the rank of physician. From what we know of him, it seems
that he was a highly skilled practitioner, but he was far more
open-minded than many of the doctors of his day and his
interest in new developments in medicine earned him the

ridicule and hostility of others who were more conservative. He was one of the first people in England to use a stethoscope and, amazing as it may seem now, this was condemned by several of the top physicians of his day who maintained that this new-fangled instrument could in no way aid diagnosis.

1828 saw the opening of the new London University and, three years later, Elliotson was appointed Professor of Medicine at University College. In 1834, he was one of the three physicians to be appointed to the new North London Hospital (renamed University College Hospital in 1837). Unfortunately, his respectable and successful career as a physician was soon to come to an end and, as with Mesmer, it was his practice of animal magnetism that caused his downfall.

He had first become interested in the subject in 1829 when he saw a demonstration given by Richard Chenevix. However, it was not until 1837 that he began to practise animal magnetism himself. In that year, he attended a series of demonstrations in which patients suffering from epilepsy were treated by Baron Dupotet, who had been working at the Salpêtrière Hospital in France, a leading centre for the treatment of diseases of the brain. He was also influenced by the theories of Franz Joseph Gall, a Viennese physician who suggested that physical disease could often be the result of the emotions acting independently of the will. However, despite his interest in the latest theories and developments in medicine, Elliotson still had deep-rooted beliefs in the magnetic fluid theory of animal magnetism and in the use of supernatural forces in the diagnosis of disease.

His own early experiments with the therapy were successful and word soon got around. Medical students began to flock to his teaching sessions. But when Elliotson began to give public demonstrations of animal magnetism, the medical staff of University College Hospital were less than pleased. And they were far from impressed by his assertion that one of his patients could, while in a trance, predict whether a person was going to die soon.

Elliotson's final fall from grace in the eyes of the orthodox medical profession was brought about by the hostility of Thomas Wakley, the founder of the medical journal the *Lancet*. Wakley had started his career as a physician and, for a time, had been a friend of Elliotson's, supporting his experiments in animal magnetism and giving his findings wide coverage in the *Lancet*. However, the two men fell out and in 1838 Wakley denounced Elliotson as a charlatan, as a result of the treatment that he had given to two sisters who suffered from epilepsy. One of these was the girl who could 'predict death' and so her case was already suspect in the eyes of the majority of the medical profession. When working with the two girls, Elliotson had used magnetized nickel, since he maintained that this metal, unlike lead, was very effective in treatment. However, Wakley discovered that these two sisters responded equally well to 'magnetic' treatment whether it was nickel or lead that was used. Since Elliotson held firmly to the theory that the treatment worked because magnetic fluid flowed through the magnetized metal plates, it seemed to Wakley that he had disproved the theory, and therefore the fact, of animal magnetism. As a result of his article, the authorities at University College Hospital were put in a very difficult position and so they asked Elliotson to stop giving demonstrations and to discharge the two sisters from the hospital. Elliotson now felt that he could no longer continue to work there and, in December of the same year, he resigned from his post.

But he did not allow the disapproval of his fellow physicians to stop him from practising the therapy in which he believed so strongly. He founded a Mesmeric Hospital in Fitzroy Square in London, and built up a large practice there. He also started his own journal, the *Zoist*, which was mainly concerned with mesmerism and which appeared quarterly for 13 years, from 1843 to 1855. Often it printed reports which the authors were unable to get published elsewhere because of hostility towards the subject matter. As a result of the *Zoist*'s influence, several centres were established around the country for the practice of mesmerism.

The use of mesmerism to control pain formed an important part of Elliotson's work. Anaesthesia was as yet unknown and patients were normally tied down and given alcohol to dull the pain of surgery. The first operation in which it is recorded that mesmerism was used was the amputation of a breast by a French surgeon, Jules Cloquet, in 1829 but it is likely that other operations had been done before this. The first operation to take place under mesmeric trance in England was the amputation of a leg performed by Drs Topham and Squire Ward in 1842. However, when the two doctors read a report of this to the Royal Medical and Chirurgical Society, they were greeted with scorn and outrage and some of the audience even suggested that the patient had been trained not to show pain. But probably the main reason why little more was heard of mesmerism in the operating theatre was the introduction, in 1846, of conventional anaesthesia.

In the same year that anaesthesia was born, Elliotson was invited to deliver the Harveian Oration, an annual lecture given by a prominent physician or surgeon. Although this was eight years after his resignation from University College Hospital and three years after he had started to publish the *Zoist*, he was obviously still well respected in the medical world. Naturally, he used the invitation as an opportunity to talk about mesmerism, which probably did not go down too well with his audience of orthodox practitioners. Over the next twenty years he managed to alienate most of the medical profession and he died in poverty in 1868.

Of the many physicians who sent accounts of their successful use of mesmerism to the *Zoist*, perhaps one of the most significant was James Esdaile. The son of a Scottish clergyman, he was born in Perth in 1808 and graduated from the University of Edinburgh in 1830. He suffered from a weak chest and, in search of warmer climes, took an appointment with the East India Company. He was sent out to India, where he was to be a surgeon at the Native Hospital at Hooghly in Bengal. In April 1845 a patient was brought in with a double hydrocoele (swelling of both sides of the scrotum). After the first side of the hydrocoele had been operated upon, the patient was in severe pain. Esdaile had read reports of Elliotson's work and knew how to induce a trance, although he had never before done so. So, in order to relieve some of the patient's pain and to allow the second part of the operation to be performed, he decided to try to mesmerize him. He thought it unlikely that he would achieve any useful results since his knowledge of mesmerism was entirely theoretical and he had never even seen anyone use it. In addition, he was dubious about the suitability of the patient, since the ideal subject was generally thought of as being a 'highly sensitive female of a nervous temperament and excitable imagination who desired to submit to the supposed influence'. However, despite his doubts, he managed to induce a trance and relieve the patient's pain, although it took him about an hour and a half. The following day, he treated the man again and, this time, induction of a trance took 45 minutes. Five days later, when the treatment was repeated for the third time, it took only 15 minutes. The native doctors who worked with Esdaile were very impressed by the results of this *belatee muntur*, or 'European charm', as they called it, and Esdaile was inspired to try it out on other patients.

Finding that the induction of a trance was often time-consuming but that the results were well worth while, he taught his native assistants how to mesmerize the patients and used his own time for performing the actual treatment. Within eight months, he had treated 18 medical cases with mesmerism, including headaches, convulsions and back pain, and had performed 73 operations on mesmerized patients, including three for cataract, the amputation of an arm and the removal of 14 scrotal tumours weighing between eight and 80 pounds. But when he wrote a report on these cases and submitted it to the Indian Medical Board, it was not even acknowledged. Having performed over a hundred operations successfully under hypnosis, he tried again and wrote another report which he sent to Sir Herbert Maddock, the Deputy Governor of Bengal. Sir Herbert was interested enough to appoint a committee, consisting of four doctors and three laymen, to investigate Esdaile's work.

The committee acknowledged that it was possible to perform painless operations on mesmerized patients but thought that the method was impractical since it took a long time to produce a deep enough trance and it was impossible to predict whether or not a patient would respond. However, Sir Herbert was sufficiently impressed by the fact that painless operations were possible to put Esdaile in charge of a small hospital in Calcutta, with five physicians and surgeons who, as 'official visitors', would report back to him. Their findings were very favourable, and they reported that patients were able to undergo major operations without pain and that post-operative shock was greatly reduced. An additional and unsolicited report was sent to the Governor General by over 300 citizens of Calcutta who had benefited from Esdaile's treatment. Finally, he was appointed as surgeon to Sarkea's Lane Hospital, where it was understood that he would combine the practice of mesmerism and orthodox medicine.

During his time in India, Esdaile performed several hundred major operations and over a thousand minor ones on mesmerized patients. Most of the major operations were to remove huge scrotal tumours which were very common in India at the time. Previously, this operation had been rarely performed because on a conscious man it had, of necessity, to be a crude and hurried affair and, as a result, about half the patients died. However, Esdaile found that with the aid of mesmerism the mortality rate dropped dramatically. While he was still in India, chloroform was introduced as an anaesthetic but Esdaile was not impressed by it since, unlike mesmerism, it had many dangers associated with it.

Unfortunately, although he submitted reports of his work to the orthodox British medical journals, Esdaile was unable to get anything published since mesmerism was still looked upon with great suspicion. There was the added difficulty that, as he was practising so far from home, no one was able to investigate his claims. But even in India his work was not accepted by the orthodox medical fraternity and none of the Indian medical journals would accept his papers. He therefore wrote a book entitled *Mesmerism in India*, which was published in 1850. In 1959, it was reissued by the Julian Press Inc. of New York under the title *Hypnosis in Medicine and Surgery*. It makes fascinating reading since it gives an account not only of Esdaile's experiences but also of his theories on mesmeric phenomena. He maintains that all that is necessary for success is 'passive obedience in the patient and a sustained attention and patience on the part of the operator'. However, he believed firmly that mesmerism was due to the transference of a 'vital fluid' from therapist to subject and, as a result, thought that some of his success was due to the fact that his patients were usually naked and had their heads shaved.

Esdaile finally left India in 1851 and returned to Scotland, writing another book (*Natural and Mesmeric Clair-voyance with the Practical Application of Mesmerism in Surgery and Medicine*) the following year. Once again he found himself unable to tolerate the cold Scottish climate and he moved to the south of England, where he died in 1859, aged 50.

Recognition of the true nature of mesmerism probably began with another Scotsman, James Braid, who was born in Fifeshire around 1795. Qualifying, like Esdaile, from Edinburgh University, he initially went into practice in Scotland but later moved to Manchester. A contemporary of both Elliotson and Esdaile, he first encountered mesmerism when, in 1841, he attended a series of demonstrations by a French practitioner, Charles de la Fontaine. His initial reaction to the display was that the man was a fraud and he actually went up on the stage with the intention of exposing him but, at close quarters, he found that the subject was indeed in a trance. He therefore started to experiment with mesmerism himself, using relatives and friends as his guinea-pigs. Following the ideas of the Abbé di Faria, he found that elaborate ritual was not necessary and that patients could be made to go into a trance simply by making them fix their eyes on a bright object. Like Esdaile, once he had become convinced of the reality of the mesmeric trance he entered wholeheartedly into its investigation, and within a month of his first encounter with it, he was lecturing on the subject. His experiments had convinced him that mesmerism was a form of sleep and he rejected completely the theory of magnetic fluids. In many ways his view of hypnosis was far more down to earth than that of some of his contemporaries and it was he who realized that the effect of the trance was to increase the patient's suggestibility.

But, despite his more rational approach, Braid, too, found himself unacceptable to orthodox medicine. In 1842, when the British Association for the Advancement of Science announced that it was to hold a meeting in Manchester, he offered to read a paper on the use of mesmerism. However, his offer was turned down. Undaunted, Braid arranged his own seminar, to coincide with the meeting of the British Association. Many members of the Association attended and saw him demonstrate his techniques. In the following year he published a book entitled *Neurypnology, or the Rationale of Nervous Sleep*, in which he described 'neuro-hypnotism or nervous sleep' as a peculiar condition of the nervous system which could be produced by the use of various techniques. As a more manageable term, he proposed the word 'hypnosis'. He denied that it was a cure for all ills but said that it would produce good or bad results according to how it was used. He maintained that only doctors should use hypnosis, warning that it was a powerful force and that those who were ignorant of how to use it correctly should not dabble with it.

Meanwhile, in Europe, interest in hypnosis had not died. Dr Ambroise-Auguste Liebeault read his first book on the subject in 1848, while he was still a medical student. Qualifying in 1850, he started up a medical practice in the French countryside and, for ten years, treated his patients by conventional methods. However, influenced by the work of James Braid, he once more started to study hypnosis and began to offer hypnotic treatment to his patients. In order to ensure that he had enough subjects, he offered this treatment free, and only charged patients to whom he gave orthodox treatment. Working in a poor rural area, he found that many of his patients were happy to take him up on the offer of free treatment and he soon had more subjects than he could cope with. In 1864 he moved to Nancy and set up a clinic devoted entirely to hypnosis where he treated patients free of charge and lived off a small private income. His medical colleagues, naturally enough, thought he was a madman.

In 1882 Liebeault cured a patient who had been suffering from sciatica for six years and whose condition Hippolyte-Marie Bernheim, Professor of Neurology at the University of Nancy, had been unable to improve. Bernheim had heard of this strange therapy being practised by Liebeault and was deeply suspicious of it. So when a report reached him about the recovery of this particular patient he went to see the hypnotherapist, determined to expose him as a charlatan. However, Liebeault was able to convince him that the mind could play an important role in the development of physical illness and that hypnosis was a valid therapy which could be used successfully in such cases. Like James Braid before him, once Bernheim had been convinced of the genuine nature of the hypnotic trance, he began to investigate the therapy with keen interest and, in 1884, he published a book entitled *De la suggestion*. In this he proposed that hypnosis produced an increased suggestibility on the part of the patient and that it was this that caused the therapist's suggestions to be effective.

Psychiatry did not become a speciality in its own right until towards the end of the nineteenth century and, before that, patients with mental disorders were often seen by neurologists. It is understandable, therefore, that Bernheim was not the only professor of neurology who became interested in hypnosis. Jean Martin Charcot (1825–93), Professor at the Salpêtrière Hospital in Paris where Mesmer's pupil Baron Dupotet had also worked, began to investigate the use of hypnosis in 1878. He was an important figure in orthodox medicine and his name is still known to physicians and surgeons today because of the many and varied conditions to which he gave his name – Charcot's biliary triad (signs by which a stone in the bile duct can be diagnosed), Charcot's intermittent hepatic fever (inflammation of the liver), Charcot's joints (painless deformed joints occurring secondary to another condition such as diabetes), Charcot–

Bouchard aneurysms (tiny weaknesses in the walls of the blood vessels of the brain) and the Charcot–Marie–Tooth syndrome (an inherited weakness of the muscles of the legs). With his obviously wide-ranging interest and ability in orthodox medicine he seems, perhaps, an unlikely candidate to have become interested in hypnosis. What is more extraordinary is that he subscribed to the theory of magnetic fluid and the use of magnets in treatment.

Charcot's main field of investigation with hypnosis was in the treatment of patients suffering from epilepsy and hysterical complaints. When treating patients whose epileptic fits were the result of a hysterical condition, he found that not only could he remove their symptoms by hypnosis but he could also bring them back again by giving the appropriate suggestions. As a result of his researches, he came to the conclusion that only patients with hysterical conditions were hypnotizable and that hypnosis itself was a form of hysteria. Since hypnosis could be used on both men and women, the corollary of Charcot's theory was that hysteria could occur in both sexes. This was a radical idea because, until then, it had been believed that hysteria was a condition that occurred only in women and that it was caused by a displacement of the womb (the word hysteria being derived from *hystera*, the Greek word for womb).

Although there was no doubt that hypnosis was particularly helpful in the treatment of patients with hysterical complaints, the idea that it was only these people who could be hypnotized was disputed by Professor Auguste Forel (1848–1931), a Swiss psychiatrist who used hypnosis on many of his patients. A great deal of work in the field of hysterical complaints was also done by the Viennese physician Dr Joseph Breuer (1842–1925) who put forward the theory that hysterical symptoms were often the result of the patient having experienced some sort of trauma. He developed the technique of regression, by which the patient could experience once again the previous trauma and, by fully expressing the emotions associated with it, get it out of his system. His work had a great influence on the young Sigmund Freud (1856–1939), with whom he worked and who, in his early years, was a keen practitioner of hypnosis. Freud qualified as a physician from the University of Vienna in 1881 and won a scholarship to undertake further studies in the department of neurology at the Salpêtrière Hospital in Paris. It was here that he met Charcot and was introduced to hypnosis and to psychology. His own use of hypnosis began in 1887 and it was this that led him to develop his own technique of psychoanalysis. It was he who coined the term 'catharsis' (from the Greek for 'cleansing') to describe the release of suppressed emotions pioneered by Breuer. Ultimately he abandoned hypnosis in favour of free association and, with the increasing interest of the medical profession in psychoanalysis, hypnosis became less and less popular in psychiatric practice.

By the end of the nineteenth century, the orthodox medical profession was beginning to thaw somewhat in its attitude towards hypnosis. In 1891 the British Medical Association set up a committee to look into the phenomena that it could produce, its value as a therapy and 'the propriety of using it'. The following year the committee produced a unanimous report in which it was agreed that the hypnotic trance was a genuine state in which might be found 'altered consciousness ... increased receptivity of suggestion from without ... an exalted condition of the attention, and post-hypnotic suggestions'. (A post-hypnotic suggestion is one which is given while the patient is in a trance and which takes effect after he has woken up.) The report commented on the fact, often re-stated since, that the term 'hypnosis' was somewhat misleading but said that the therapy itself was often effective in 'relieving pain, procuring sleep and alleviating many functional ailments'.

It pointed out that dangers might occur as the result of 'want of knowledge, carelessness or intentional abuse' and reiterated James Braid's recommendation, made 50 years earlier, that only doctors should be allowed to practise the therapy. It also expressed strong disapproval of public exhibitions of hypnotism and recommended that these should be restricted by law. However, despite the continuing concern of doctors, public exhibitions of hypnotism are still allowed nearly a hundred years later.

During the First World War, a large number of casualties suffering from shell shock, together with a shortage of Army psychiatrists, produced a situation in which the latter were happy to use anything that would speed up the patient's recovery. This led to a resurgence of interest in hypnosis. But practitioners were now beginning to find other uses for hypnosis in addition to the treatment of purely psychiatric complaints. Its use for dental extractions, in place of anaesthesia, was probably pioneered by a Scot, James Milne Bramwell (1852–1925), who worked in the Midlands. His interest in hypnosis had started when he was a child living in Perth. His father, Dr J. P. Bramwell, had seen demonstrations given by Esdaile, who at that time was working in the same city, and his enthusiasm had communicated itself to young James. In time, James followed his father into the medical profession and, while training at Edinburgh University, was particularly interested by a part of the physiology course which the Professor, John Hughes Bennett, devoted to the work of James Braid. Once qualified, he went into general practice and started to use hypnosis for himself. In 1890, at a meeting in Leeds, he demonstrated hypnotic anaesthesia to a medical audience. Both the *British Medical Journal* and the *Lancet* carried reports of the meeting and, as a result, Bramwell had so many patients sent to him that he had to abandon his general practice and concentrate solely on hypnosis.

It was the use of hypnosis as an anaesthetic that made it so useful in dental treatment where, for minor procedures, a general anaesthetic seemed unwarranted. On some occasions Bramwell was present and hypnotized the patient before the dentist started work. But for some patients this was unnecessary and for these he would use the technique of post-hypnotic suggestion, telling them that, when they were in the dentist's chair, if a certain phrase should be repeated to them they would immediately go into a deep hypnotic trance. Then all he had to do was to write to the patient's dentist, telling him which phrase to use, and the patient could be hypnotized every time he went for dental treatment.

However, dentists proved to be as hard to convince as physicians had been and it was a long time before the use of hypnosis in dentistry became acceptable to more than just a few. The first sign that attitudes were slowly changing was probably the publication, in 1938, of a paper on the subject by the *British Dental Journal* – the journal of orthodox dentistry. The author of the paper, Eric Wookey, suggested that hypnosis could be of use to remove pain during scaling, fillings, extractions and minor oral surgery, and that it would also help to alleviate fear and pain experienced before the treatment began. He had, he said, convincing evidence that hypnosis could be of real value and he thought it was a strong possibility that it could also promote rapid healing and prevent haemorrhage, although proof of this was harder to obtain. By writing the article he hoped to induce his colleagues to take up the study of hypnosis so that their combined experiences could be put together for the benefit of the dental profession. However, it was another 14 years before this was followed up. Then, in 1952, an Essex dentist, Harry Radin, proposed the setting up of a committee of dentists to study hypnosis. Eric Wookey was appointed Chairman and the committee itself evolved into the British Society of Dental Hypnosis.

By this time, more interest had been aroused within the medical profession and the top medical hypnotherapists of the day were sharing their expertise by writing papers for the *Journal of Hypnosis*, which had been founded in 1949 by Dr S. J. Van Pelt. Sadly, although Van Pelt was able to bring together in this way the top names in hypnosis, he met with hostility from the orthodox medical profession and detailed proposals that he made for teaching hypnotherapy to doctors were not taken up.

The founding of the British Society of Dental Hypnosis in 1952 was the signal for a sudden burst of publicity for dental hypnosis. It started when a demonstration of a dental extraction under hypnosis at the annual meeting of the British Dental Association was reported widely and in extravagant terms by journalists who still equated hypnosis with entertainment and mumbo jumbo. Only two weeks later, the BBC television programme *Panorama* showed another dental extraction under hypnosis, which resulted in even greater press coverage.

In 1953, a sub-group of the Psychological Medicine Group Committee of the British Medical Association was appointed to look into the use of hypnosis in medicine. It reported that the sort of phenomena that occurred under hypnosis shed a great deal of light on the workings of the unconscious mind. It found that hypnosis was of use in surgery, obstetrics and dentistry and suggested that it might be the treatment of choice for some psychosomatic and psychiatric illnesses. It recommended, therefore, that medical students should learn about hypnosis as part of their psychiatric training and that courses should be available for anaesthetists and obstetricians. But, 34 years later, hypnosis is still taught mainly in post-graduate courses and is a closed book to many anaesthetists and obstetricians.

It was not until the early 1960s that the press began to report on the practice of hypnotherapy in terms that recognized its scientific basis and its valuable practical applications. But within the medical profession, interest was growing. The British Society of Dental Hypnosis had, in 1955, become the Dental and Medical Society for the Study of Hypnosis and, in 1961, when it amalgamated with a group of doctors who were practising hypnosis, it was renamed the Society for Medical and Dental Hypnosis. In 1968 this became the British Society for Medical and Dental Hypnosis and it continues its work today under this name. Nowadays there are satellite groups of doctors and dentists around the country, running and attending courses on different aspects of hypnotherapy. Courses are run for doctors and dentists who are interested in learning something about the subject or who wish to train in order to be able to use hypnotherapy as part of their practice. Meetings are held with societies in other parts of the world under the auspices of the European Society of Hypnosis and the International Society of Hypnosis, and eminent specialists from other countries are brought over to speak at conferences. The medical hypnotherapist of today is a far cry from Mesmer and, with the abandoning of the 'mystical' aspect of hypnosis, the therapy has become a respected medical tool.

CHAPTER THREE

PSYCHOSOMATIC ILLNESS:

THE EFFECT OF THE MIND

ON THE BODY

As the practice of hypnotherapy has developed, it has become clear that it is of value in the treatment of many different conditions. These may be divided roughly into three groups: those in which there is need for pain control (for example, dentistry and obstetrics), those in which the condition is purely a mental one (such as the phobias), and those in which the patient is suffering from a psychosomatic disorder. Now, 'psychosomatic' is a greatly misunderstood word, since people often believe it to mean that the disease is all in the mind or that the symptoms are being imagined by the patient. But someone who is suffering from a psychosomatic disorder knows full well that his symptoms are real. The patient who *imagines* that he is ill is a hypochondriac – something quite different.

A psychosomatic disease is one in which the mind affects the body to such an extent that the body becomes physically ill. The word is derived from two Greek words – *psyche* ('mind') and *soma* ('body'), and the implication is that both are equally involved. Hypnotherapy, of course, only treats the mind but is effective because psychosomatic illness can be either caused or made worse by certain mental states. Therefore if one can treat the precipitating or aggravating mental cause – usually anxiety or stress – the bodily component has a better chance of getting better because it is no longer being 'fed' by the mental component.

For example, it is well known that people who have very stressful jobs have an increased tendency to develop duodenal ulcers. No one would suggest that a duodenal ulcer is 'all in the mind', but there is no doubt that if the patient had been under less stress he might have been able to avoid developing the ulcer. Anxiety and stress have the effect of making the stomach secrete an excess of digestive acid which eats away at the lining of the duodenum (the first part of the small bowel, into which the stomach contents flow), causing ulceration. Medication may reduce the acidity and therefore control the ulcer but is only likely to cure it if the stress is removed. One can compare the situation to that of a bath with the taps left running. When it starts to overflow, one may be able to keep the floor dry by means of vigorous use of a mop and bucket – but the only sure way of preventing a flood is to turn the taps off. Thus, in the case of a patient with an ulcer, if the precipitating stress continues, simple medical therapy may not be able to cure it and ultimately he may require surgery.

Similarly, patients who have recurrent asthma often find that an attack occurs if they become distressed or anxious. The attack is genuine enough but the precipitating cause is a mental one. And because asthma is such a frightening condition, the patient's anxiety may increase dramatically when he starts having difficulty in breathing. Thus a vicious circle is set up with the asthmatic attack and the anxiety feeding on each other. If the patient is taught a method by which he can avoid anxiety, he is likely to have fewer and less severe attacks.

As well as being able to make the body do things that are unwanted, the mind can also prevent the body from performing functions that the patient actually wants it to. Most men have, at one time or another, been unable to achieve an erection. It may be because they are tired or have had too much alcohol. Whatever the cause, it is likely that it will no longer be affecting them the next time they try to have intercourse. Many men realize this and accept the temporary failure as just that – temporary. However, sometimes a man – perhaps unable to understand why he should have failed on this particular occasion – will start to worry about it. The next time he wants to have sex, there will be a nagging anxiety in the back of his mind that he may not be able to get an erection. And, if the anxiety becomes too great, this in itself may prevent him from having an erection. Finally he may become impotent entirely as a result of his anxiety about impotence and for no other reason. In this case, if the patient can stop worrying about getting an erection (helped perhaps by hypnotherapy or psychosexual counselling), then he should be able to get back to normal again.

Why is it, then, that the body can be so affected by the mind? Is it that we persuade ourselves that we are ill and then become so? No, not at all. It's all due to the fact that the body and the mind are *not* separate entities living in different worlds but are fully integrated parts of the whole patient. Unfortunately, Western medicine is inclined to divide the patient up and treat him as though he were a loose collection of relatively unconnected parts: if he has a mental illness he sees a psychiatrist, if he has arthritis he sees a rheumatologist, if he has appendicitis he sees a surgeon. However, in recent years the concept of holism, which underlies most of the complementary therapies, has started to find a place in orthodox medicine. A practitioner of holistic medicine treats the whole patient, not his individual parts (the term is derived from the Greek word *holos* meaning 'whole'). If the patient comes complaining of, for example, arthritis, the holistic practitioner will wish to know not only about the patient's joints but also about how the rest of his body functions, his state of mind and any anxieties he may have, his job and the stresses it puts on him, his home life, his social life, what he eats, what exercise he gets, his hopes and ambitions, his sleeping patterns and so on. These are all things that make up that individual patient and, if he is ill, they may all contribute to that illness or be affected by it.

In order to understand why it is that the body and the mind can interact to such an extent that the mind can cause physical illness, we must look, briefly, at the way in which they work. If one studies the anatomy of the human body, it soon becomes clear that, although different parts may seem totally unlike each other (for example, the kidneys and the tongue or the lungs and the feet) there are two things that they all have in common. In order to remain alive and functioning, every part of the body (apart from those which are made of a dead substance, such as the fingernails and the hair) has to have a blood supply and a nerve supply. The blood supply is controlled by the heart, which pumps the blood around the body. The brain does not control the nervous system in quite the same way, although it is the most complex part of that system and must be thought of as its centre. It is responsible for all the 'higher' functions, such as thinking, memory, speech, hearing and sight. But many simpler functions are carried out through the extension of the brain, the spinal cord, which runs down the back, inside the hard protective cover of the bones of the spine, or vertebrae. This is why it is possible for a person with a broken back to be paralysed although the brain is undamaged, and why people with severe brain damage may still retain some normal bodily functions.

Both brain and spinal cord are made up of very delicate tissue and both have to be protected – the brain within the skull and the spinal cord within the vertebral column. However, in order to function, nerves have to leave this protected environment and run out into the rest of the body, where they can receive messages and send back signals which tell the body how to function. This 'exterior' part of the system is known as the peripheral nervous system, while the brain and spinal cord form the central nervous system. The head, its special sense organs (eye, ear, nose and tongue) and the neck are supplied by nerves which come directly from the brain and leave it through little holes in the skull. These nerves coming from the brain are known as the cranial nerves and one of them, the vagus, travels further than the others and plays an important role in the function of the throat and voice, the stomach, intestines, heart and lungs. The spinal column itself is made up of small bones or vertebrae which are jointed together, allowing us to move and bend. Where a vertebra joins its neighbour, two nerves leave the spinal cord, one going to the right side of the body, the other to the left. Thus, the whole of the body is supplied by these nerves, which divide and divide to form a huge network.

Although one thinks of individual nerves as being continuous, solid cords, they are, in fact, made up of many tiny fibres which interact with each other. It is rather like a piece of rope which can be pulled to pieces to reveal the thousands of tiny fibres which make it up. When a message is passed down a nerve, it takes the form of an electrical impulse. However, where two nerve fibres meet, there is a tiny gap across which the impulse cannot pass. When it reaches the end of a fibre, therefore, it causes a chemical to be released which stimulates the next fibre to pass the electrical impulse along its length. It is through control of the various chemicals that nerve endings produce (the 'neurotransmitters') that modern medicine has gained some of its control of the nervous system. For example, some of the muscle relaxants that are used on patients undergoing major operations act by preventing the release of a neurotransmitter which passes on a message telling muscles to contract. Therefore, although the nervous system can be thought of in terms of an electric circuit or a telephone switchboard, it is, in fact, very much more intricate than either of these.

In terms of function, the nervous system is divided into two sections, the somatic, or voluntary, and the autonomic, or involuntary. (We have already met the word 'somatic', meaning 'bodily', in the term 'psychosomatic'). The autonomic nervous system, as its alternative name implies, functions automatically and is in charge of all the body functions that one does not have to think about consciously, whereas the somatic nervous system is concerned with voluntary action. For example, to move your arm or your leg, you must have a conscious wish to do so. It doesn't just happen – you don't suddenly find yourself walking down the street when you want to be sitting down reading a book. In other words, you have control of such functions as moving, talking and so on. However, you don't have control over basic bodily functions such as the beating of your heart and your breathing. Although it is possible to control the muscles of the chest that are involved in breathing, and therefore to hold your breath for a short while, you can't do it indefinitely. And you don't have to remember to keep breathing, you do it automatically. Similarly, your blood keeps circulating and your food gets digested even if you're busy thinking of other things.

Obviously it is essential that these functions should occur automatically, or we'd none of us live very long and, while we were alive, we would have very little time for thinking of anything other than keeping our lungs, hearts and digestive systems working. However, because all these things do happen automatically, it follows that we have very little control over them and have to trust our autonomic nervous systems to keep them functioning normally. If you bend your leg and it hurts your knee to do so, then it's a relatively simple procedure to unbend it again to relieve the pain. However, if, for example, the autonomic nervous system starts to cause excessive production of acid in the stomach, it's less easy to get it back to normal.

The autonomic nervous system itself is divided into two sections, the sympathetic and the parasympathetic, and, in a healthy person, these two will balance each other, since they work in opposite directions. Thus the heart will beat neither too slowly nor too fast, the stomach will produce the correct amount of acid in order to digest the food that is presented to it and breathing will continue at a normal rate. However, there is a reason why we have two opposing systems regulating these basic body functions rather than just one. Every now and again our bodies need to do something which is not normal in order to adapt to changing circumstances and to protect themselves from danger. This function is performed by the sympathetic nervous system, which originally developed so that we could protect ourselves from predators and other dangers, a role that it still plays in animals. However, although human beings are seldom threatened nowadays by man-eating tigers or fierce cavemen, the system continues to work in exactly the same way if we happen to be faced with anything that seems threatening. This can include a multitude of situations – for example, an interview for a job, an examination, stage fright, driving a car in heavy traffic, meeting a large spider, or seeing a traffic warden bearing down on your parked car when you've left it on a double yellow line. The dangers faced by people in the Western world are, on the whole, far less life-threatening than those which faced primitive man, but we still react with the same 'fight or flight' response. Thus, when confronted with a traffic warden or a job interview, our bodies react as though it were necessary for us to fight or to turn on our heels and run. These reactions may be totally inappropriate to the situation, but this is the way the body still works.

When the sympathetic nervous system is stimulated, the pupils of the eyes widen, the tiny muscles attached to the base of each hair contract so that the hair stands on end (very useful if you're a small animal trying to pretend that you're bigger and fiercer than you really are), the heart rate speeds up (so that the body is supplied with as much oxygen as possible), the arteries supplying blood to the heart dilate so that the heart can work harder, and the muscles in the bronchial tubes relax so that air can go in and out rapidly and easily. In addition, blood is diverted away from the digestive tract and other functions that, for the time being, are not essential and is sent to the limbs to assist speedy running away. This is done by constricting the blood vessels of the former and dilating those that supply the latter. If there is considerable dilation of the blood vessels in the limbs but running away is not appropriate to the situation (for example, when you are confronted by a traffic warden), then the blood pressure may suddenly drop. (If one did run away, the exercise would maintain the blood pressure at a normal level.) A sudden drop in blood pressure may reduce the supply of blood to the brain and one may faint. This is why it is possible to faint as the result of a severe shock. In addition to all these reactions, stimulation of the sympathetic nervous system causes the sweat glands to release sweat and the adrenal glands to release adrenaline.

The hormone adrenaline is produced by the medulla, or inside section, of the adrenal glands which lie, one on each side, on top of the kidneys. It is responsible for many of the reactions that occur in response to fright or shock. When the emotion is a happy one – excitement rather than fright – the sensation of a 'surge of adrenaline' can be quite a pleasant one. Even when it is less pleasant, it can be helpful. Even the top professional actors and singers admit to having 'nerves' before going on stage and know that the adrenaline that is responsible helps to keep them on their toes so that they can give a first-rate performance. The 'nerves' normally disappear as soon as a performer steps on stage but, if he has been feeling frightened, rather than nervous and excited, he may produce far more adrenaline than he needs; as a result, he may still feel nervous once he's performing and so may give less than his best. It's exactly the same with exam nerves – the student who is slightly nervous and 'keyed up' beforehand is likely to do better than either the student who has no emotions or the one who is very agitated.

But, of course, the original function of adrenaline was not to help us to perform well on stage or to pass exams. It was to prepare the body for fight or flight. Like all hormones, it is secreted directly from the gland into the blood stream and is carried to all the organs of the body, where it acts to reinforce the responses resulting from the stimulation of the sympathetic nervous system. It also acts on the liver, causing it to release stored glucose, raising the blood glucose level and thus supplying the energy needed for running or fighting.

The 'flight or fight' response is, of course, an emergency one. We are not built to be in a constant state of stimulation and yet, nowadays, that is the way that many of us live. An animal living in the wild will have its autonomic nervous system stimulated perhaps three or four times a day, maybe more, when it is tracking and killing prey or when it is being tracked and is having to fight. But in between these episodes it will be in a relaxed state during which its nervous system can go back to normal. Not so with human beings. We are constantly stimulating our bodies with stressful jobs, driving in heavy traffic, watching horror movies, listening to the news, arguing with family and friends, getting involved in politics – the list goes on and on. And as if this were not enough, excessive secretion of adrenaline or other hormones can also be caused by eating large amounts of sugar and 'junk' foods, drinking coffee and alcohol, and smoking. And all the time that we are doing this, our autonomic nervous systems are having to try to cope and keep our bodies functioning normally. Little wonder, then, that stress, anxiety, smoking and bad eating and drinking habits can lead to illness. The body may react in one of two ways: it may be in a constant state of sympathetic-type anxiety (i.e., ready to fight or fly); or the symptoms may be those of parasympathetic over-activity, which may sometimes occur if the sympathetic system has been exhausted by an excess of stimulants and, as a result, become underactive.

An imbalance between two parts of the autonomic nervous system is at the root of many psychosomatic diseases. For example, a peptic ulcer, in which excessive gastric juices are produced, may be associated with excessive parasympathetic stimulation, as may asthma, in which the muscles in the bronchial tubes contract down and thus narrow the airways in the lungs. Migraine is thought to be due to the blood vessels of the brain first contracting and then dilating, functions which are controlled by the opposing parts of the autonomic nervous system. Similarly, irritable bowel syndrome occurs when the large bowel ceases to function normally and is either overactive or underactive, leading to episodes of diarrhoea interspersed with episodes of constipation. One important thing that these diseases have in common is that they all get worse if the patient is tense, anxious or upset. Even happy excitement may cause symptoms to arise. It is not uncommon to hear a patient with irritable bowel syndrome complaining that he had to miss some event that he was looking forward to because he had a sudden attack of diarrhoea. There are other conditions, too, such as eczema and psoriasis, that get worse when the patient is upset or worried, although they cannot be quite so readily explained in terms of the autonomic nervous system.

It will be obvious that, in the case of diseases associated with an imbalance of the autonomic nervous system, if one can prevent abnormal stimulation of that system, one should be able to control the disease. And in order to prevent abnormal stimulation one must, of course, eat and drink sensibly, stop smoking and remain calm. Eating and drinking sensibly may be done by most people without too much effort. Even stopping smoking is often not as difficult as it might appear. But to remain calm if you have a naturally anxious temperament may seem like a hopeless task. However, this is where hypnotherapy can help because it is, first and foremost, a very effective relaxation technique. When you go into hypnosis your body – and your mind – suddenly discover that it is possible for them to relax. Suggestions are then given, while you are in hypnosis, that you will be less tense and less anxious while you're going about your everyday life and, as a result, you will be able to contribute a great deal towards keeping in control whichever problem it is that is affecting you. Thus hypnotherapy is widely used for the treatment of asthma, migraine and irritable bowel syndrome and may contribute towards the satisfactory healing of a peptic ulcer. It may also help to clear up other conditions, such as eczema and psoriasis, which get worse when the patient is anxious. Psychosomatic illness can be seen as a vicious circle of which anxiety is a vital component. Removing the anxiety will break the circle and allow the body's own defence mechanisms which, up till then, have been fighting a losing battle, to take over and restore the patient to health.

Even today, no one is entirely sure how hypnosis works in relation to the brain and nervous system. Little wonder, then, that the ideas of animal magnetism remained popular for so long. Dr Peter Mellett (in the *Proceedings* of the British Society of Medical and Dental Hypnosis, January 1981) describes hypnosis as 'an unusual or altered state of consciousness in which distortions of perception occur as uncritical responses of the subject to notions from an objective source (the hypnotist) or a subjective source (his own memory) or both'. In other words, the patient is open to suggestions that things are different from the way they really are and he will accept these suggestions uncritically. So a patient who is in pain can be told that his pain is going and he may indeed feel it disappearing. Or, as sometimes happens in stage hypnosis, a subject is handed a piece of apple and told that it is an onion, and his eyes start to water just as though he were smelling an onion. In other words, his autonomic nervous system, which controls automatic reactions such as crying, is responding to what the subject believes. It is, so to speak, the other side of the coin from the man who cannot get an erection because he believes it will not happen and therefore it doesn't; the man with the phoney onion believes it will make his eyes water and therefore it does.

Some experiments done on allergic subjects show how very strongly our beliefs affect the way in which our bodies react. If a patient has a small amount of a substance to which he is allergic (known as an allergen) injected into the skin of his forearm, the skin will react by producing a red raised patch around the site of the injection. This technique is commonly used in skin clinics to try to find out which particular substances a patient is allergic to. In the experiments, patients who were known to react to certain allergens were injected with them while under hypnosis. They were told what they were being injected with and, sure enough, they reacted just as they would have if awake. Then they were injected in the opposite arm with a small amount of sterile water. They were told that this was a substance to which they were not allergic and therefore they would not react – and, of course, they didn't. So far, it all seems perfectly straightforward and what one would expect. However, when the reaction had settled, the patients were hypnotized again and, once more, were injected with an allergen in one arm and sterile water in the other. Only this time they were told that the allergen was the water and the water the allergen. And, extraordinary as it may seem, they reacted to the water and didn't react to the allergen. In another experiment, patients were injected in both arms with the identical allergen, but were told that only one of the injections contained the allergen and that the other was water. And they reacted only in the one arm which they thought had been injected with the allergen. Thus the mind can control the autonomic nervous system to such an extent that it is capable of allowing tiny blood vessels to dilate and fluid to seep out of them (as happens in an allergic reaction) in an area of skin that may be no more than a centimetre across.

Experiments such as these show very clearly the effect of hypnosis on the automatic functions of the body. But how the hypnotic state actually occurs is more difficult to say. There appear to be no signs that a patient is in hypnosis. A patient who is asleep, for example, may have a slower heart rate than normal and may breathe more slowly and deeply. His blood pressure may drop and an electro-encephalogram (EEG or) 'trace' of his brain waves will show a pattern of slow waves interspersed with faster spikes, the latter being associated with periods of rapid eye movement and dreaming. A patient who is unconscious will also show changes in his heart and breathing rate, his blood pressure and his EEG, the changes depending on the reason for his unconsciousness (for example, the changes seen in a patient in diabetic coma would not necessarily be the same as those seen in someone who had concussion). But in a patient who is in hypnosis there seem to be no specific changes. His heart rate and respiration rate may slow down and his blood pressure drop, but not necessarily any more than in someone who is just sitting in a chair, completely relaxed. And the EEG will show the same pattern as if he were awake. While he is going into hypnosis, it will show the slow wave patterns that occur if one sits quietly with eyes shut and thinks of nothing. When the hypnotherapist starts to talk to him and make suggestions for him to think about, the EEG will show that the brain is thinking, as in someone who is awake. It is for this reason, perhaps, that some people have found it very difficult to accept that there is such a state as hypnosis, and yet patients who have been in hypnosis and therapists who have seen what can be done with hypnosis have no doubt.

Normally the brain is open to all sorts of stimuli. It receives messages from the eyes and interprets them so that we see, and it translates the stimuli that reach the ears into different sounds; it receives information about smell, taste, feeling and the position of the body, and it is aware of pain. It has been suggested by some researchers that, in hypnosis, when the patient is made to concentrate on a single thing, the brain becomes less aware of the input coming from the other senses. The continuous, monotonous speech of the hypnotist could then lull the brain until all it was aware of was this speech. Thus the speech would assume a very important role, since it would not have to compete for the brain's attention with the usual input coming from the eyes, the nose, the tongue and the rest of the body.

However, how can one explain the fact that while under hypnosis the patient's subconscious mind is so much more readily accessible than normal? This, after all, is the reason why post-hypnotic suggestions work – they are planted in the subconscious and the patient obeys them automatically, without having to think about them. In addition, the subconscious can reveal what is troubling it far more readily and old suppressed memories and emotions can be brought to the fore and dealt with.

It has been suggested by a number of investigators that these effects of hypnosis are due to the differences in function of the left and the right sides of the brain. The two sides of the brain are, to all intents and purposes, identical in structure, with the right side receiving messages from the left side of the body and the left side receiving messages from the right. This is why, if someone has a stroke caused by a blood clot occurring in the right side of his brain, the resultant paralysis will affect the left side of his body; if the left side of his brain is affected, then the right side of his body will be paralysed. However, if the paralysis is on the right (and the damage on the left), he is far more likely to find that his speech is affected than if the paralysis is on the left. This is because the two sides of the brain do not function in exactly the same way. The left hemisphere is concerned with speech and logical thinking. The right hemisphere, however, has a very limited function in speech but is more concerned with emotions and intuition. Experiments have shown that the right hemisphere can recognize things but cannot put a name to them. Therefore a patient whose right hemisphere is functioning alone will know what to do with a knife and fork but will accept uncritically the information that they are called 'a cup and saucer'.

These discoveries have led to the theory that, when a patient is under hypnosis, the logical left side of his brain relaxes and allows the right side to come to the fore. This would explain the ability of the patient, under hypnosis, to bring out long-repressed memories (the repression being a function of the left side of the brain) and to accept uncritically suggestions that are put to him, since these will not seem to be illogical.

CHAPTER FOUR

HYPNOSIS IN THERAPY

AND ON THE STAGE

There is no doubt that most people who have been hypnotized find it a very pleasant and relaxing experience. Indeed, many are reluctant to come out of the hypnotic state at the end of their session, in the same way that they might be reluctant to wake up from a pleasant dream in a warm bed when they know they have a busy day ahead.

Before waking a patient out of hypnosis, a therapist will usually tell him that when he comes out of the trance he will feel relaxed, happy, content, free of pain, or whatever is appropriate to the situation. So the patient, who has been sitting in an extremely relaxed state for half an hour or so, may start to feel the benefit of the treatment as soon as he opens his eyes. With some patients this benefit is only small at first. But others may say that they feel that a weight has been lifted from their shoulders or that they are feeling more relaxed than they have done for a long time.

However, it must be stressed that a patient has got to want to get better in order for hypnotherapy to be able to help him, since it is, first and foremost, a self-help therapy. It will help the patient to do what, in his heart of hearts, he wants to do. There may, however, be reasons why he does not want his condition to improve, which are rooted in his subconscious mind and may therefore be quite unknown to him. In such a case, he is unlikely to feel much benefit from his sessions unless, somehow, this unwillingness to get better can be discovered and brought out during hypnosis. It may seem strange that there are patients who want to remain ill, but this may happen, for example, if the patient has done something for which, subconsciously, he cannot forgive himself and for which he is punishing himself, or if he is gaining actual benefit from his illness, such as increased attention or not having to face up to responsibilities. The latter case, which is known as secondary gain, must be distinguished from that of the malingerer who feigns illness in order to gain an advantage. In secondary gain, the illness is quite real and stems from an attitude of the subconscious mind. The majority of patients, fortunately, have no such problems and are anxious to get better, so that for these the hypnotherapy session is a comfortable and relaxed period after which they may feel a definite benefit.

Patients who are considering having hypnotherapy are often dubious as to whether they would be 'good subjects' and it may be this doubt that puts many of them off trying it. Obviously, if you don't think that you can be hypnotized, then there is little point in going to a hypnotherapist. However, it is fairly rare for people to be completely unhypnotizable and many patients are amazed at how readily they 'go under', even at the first session. In fact, most people have been in a light hypnotic trance many times in their lives. The commonest way of going into hypnosis by oneself is to daydream. Most people know what it is like to go into a vivid daydream, where one loses all sense of time and of one's actual surroundings. And when one wakes up from the daydream, it is sometimes a shock to find that it was not real and that one is not in the place that one was imagining. This vivid kind of daydream is a form of hypnosis and it can be understood, therefore, why people with vivid imaginations are usually good hypnotic subjects – they have had lots of experience!

Hypnosis and Meditation

Some types of meditation also induce a form of hypnotic state, particularly those, such as Transcendental Meditation, in which a word or phrase (*mantra*) is repeated over and over again. This is a meditation technique which many people have found helpful in relieving anxieties and tension, in making them more positive in outlook and in clearing up conditions related to anxiety such as eczema and irritable bowel syndrome.

It would be wrong, however, to assume that all forms of meditation induce a hypnotic state in those who practise them. The term 'meditation' can mean different things to different people, meditation techniques are many and varied and some are completely unrelated to hypnosis. For example, in the Buddhist system of mindfulness of breathing, although the practitioner concentrates on the breath going in and out, his aim is not to concentrate on that to the exclusion of all else but to focus the mind so perfectly that he is aware of everything that is going on around him.

An interesting distinction between this form of meditation and hypnosis has been made by some healers who have observed the different effects of each upon the aura, or psychic energy, of the individual. The purpose of Buddhist and various other forms of meditation is to increase the spiritual awareness of the practitioner and those who can see auras say that they do, in fact, grow larger in those who meditate regularly, being particularly noticeable during the act of meditation. (Legend says that the Buddha had an aura three miles wide!) But when a patient is put into hypnosis, his aura retracts inwards. In other words, the psychic energy and the 'higher functions' of the mind are temporarily shut down, while the deeper, subconscious mind becomes opened up.

More scientifically, the differences between meditation

to increase spiritual awareness, the 'hypnotic' forms of meditation, and hypnosis itself may be demonstrated by wiring a subject up to an E E G (electro-encephalograph or brain wave) machine. A subject who is sitting, relaxed, with his eyes shut, or who is in hypnosis, or who is practising a 'hypnotic' form of meditation will show on the E E G a pattern of slow waves, known as 'alpha' waves, interspersed with rapid so-called 'beta' waves which appear when he is spoken to or when he is asked to think about something. A constantly repeated short noise will produce, to begin with, a short burst of beta waves each time it is heard, but after a time the brain will grow accustomed to the sound and will, apparently, stop hearing it, since it no longer registers on the E E G. However, with some forms of meditation the result is quite different. William Johnston, in his book *Silent Music* (Collins Fount Paperbacks, 1974), describes an experiment in which experienced Zen meditators were put onto E E G machines. It was found that they never grew accustomed to anything – each time they heard something, their brains reacted as though they were hearing it for the very first time.

However, the effect of Transcendental Meditation on the brain seems, from these experiments with E E Gs, to be very similar to that of hypnosis. It follows, therefore, that someone who is used to doing this kind of meditation and who had found benefit from it is likely to find hypnotherapy helpful. But familiarity with other forms of meditation will not necessarily make one a good hypnotic subject. As I have mentioned, patients who have vivid daydreams or who are very imaginative are usually very susceptible to hypnosis, but it is said that some of the best subjects are nurses, actors and members of the armed forces, because they are used to taking orders or directions from other people. Actors have the additional advantage of being imaginative as well.

The Depth of the Trance

The difference between the sort of hypnotic trance which is induced by daydreaming or by chanting a mantra and that which is induced by a hypnotherapist is that the former is just a light trance and no more, whereas the latter can be used to produce more effects than simply those of relaxation. Of course, in a self-induced trance one can give oneself instructions and directions, but somehow they don't seem to have the same force as those given by someone else in whom one has trust. Patients who are taught self-hypnosis, for practice at home, often say that, although pleasant, it doesn't seem to have the same quality as a trance induced by the therapist.

Patients are usually aware of how deep a trance is and can feel themselves going deeper. There are, in fact, techniques that can be used by the therapist to estimate the depth of the patient's trance. However, these require some concentration on the part of the patient and, since this may lighten the trance, they are not often used. One such technique, which is known as the Lecron rating, requires the patient to visualize a scale of nought to a hundred – something like a very large thermometer – and to picture a needle somewhere along the scale indicating the depth of his trance, with nought indicating a wide-awake state and one hundred indicating the deepest trance that he has ever been in. If a patient is asked to do this repeatedly, his rating is likely to approach nearer and nearer to nought as the concentration required each time progressively lightens his trance.

Some patients are concerned because they feel that they don't go very deeply into trance, but this usually doesn't matter very much. There are some forms of treatment, such as age regression, where a deep trance is essential in order to achieve results, and certainly patients do seem to respond better to suggestions if they are in a deeper trance, but this does not mean to say that one cannot treat a patient who can only achieve a light trance. Indeed, there is plenty of treatment that can be carried out with only a very light trance and, although the condition may take longer to resolve if the patient can never achieve anything deeper, it is still perfectly possible to have good results from hypnotherapy. Patients should not worry, therefore, about whether or not they are 'good subjects'. It is the results of the treatment that are important, not the depth of the trance.

The Hypnotherapy Session

A first session with a hypnotherapist will usually last about an hour (unless the patient is being treated to stop smoking, in which case it may be shorter). The therapist will take a full case history and will want to know not just about the complaint itself but also about the patient's attitude to it and whether anything makes the symptoms worse or better. He will need details of the patient's home circumstances, his job, his lifestyle and any anxieties or worries that he may have. There are two reasons why the therapist needs to know such a lot about his patient: firstly to help him discover the cause of the trouble, and secondly so that, when giving post-hypnotic suggestions, he can express himself in terms that will be readily accepted by the patient. For example, if a migraine-sufferer says that his attack always starts with little dots of yellow light swimming in front of his eyes and that he then gets a numb feeling in his mouth, the therapist can tell him, when he is in hypnosis, that these specific symptoms will not occur. This is far more effective than just telling him that he will not get migraine. Similarly, if a patient finds something helpful –

perhaps a cream to stop a skin condition from irritating –
he can be told that performing a certain action (taking a
deep breath, perhaps) will relieve the itching in exactly the
same way that the cream does. Thus the patient has something within his own experience to which he can relate the
therapist's suggestion and therefore it is more likely to be
effective.

Very often, on the first occasion that they are hypnotized
patients only achieve a light trance. This may be because
they are still slightly apprehensive about the therapy or
anxious that they may prove to be unhypnotizable. By the
second session, these anxieties will have dispersed and the
patient is likely to be more relaxed and receptive to the
treatment. The techniques that are used to induce a trance
are many and varied and different practitioners have their
own favourites. Usually they are fairly simple, but the
techniques beloved by film-makers of the swinging fob
watch, or the 'look into my eyes – you are falling asleep'
muttered in a foreign accent, are seldom used!

Once the patient has gone into a trance, the therapist will
use various methods to deepen it. A popular one is to ask
the patient to imagine that he is walking in a beautiful
garden and gradually everything in the garden becomes
very clear so that he can see the individual flowers, smell
the roses and hear the birds singing. This is just an extension of the 'vivid daydream' mentioned earlier. Being
able to lose himself in a daydream like this will, of itself,
make the patient more relaxed and allow the trance to
deepen. However, another deepening technique can be used
in conjunction with it. For example, the therapist may ask
the patient to picture some steps going down to a lower
level of the garden; as he sees himself walking slowly down
these steps, the trance gradually becomes deeper and
deeper.

Imagining downward movement is a very effective way

of deepening a trance and, for those patients who do not suffer from claustrophobia and who do not mind travelling in lifts, visualizing a downward journey in a lift can increase the depth considerably. One method is to tell the patient that the lift is descending from about the fifth floor, and that at each floor the lift stops and a certain number of people get in and get out, so that each journey from floor to floor acts as a separate deepening technique. Finally, the lift goes down into the basement – 'the basement of relaxation' – and the patient gets out and moves into a warm, softly lit room, where he sinks down into a comfortable chair. However, the therapist really needs to have his wits about him if he is using this method, or the patient may finish up no deeper in trance than at the start. One therapist tells of an occasion when he used this technique, saying, 'We are now at the fourth floor and two people get out and one gets in . . . we are now at the third floor and one person gets out and one gets in . . .' and so on, without concentrating on the numbers he was using. It seemed to him when he had finished that the patient wasn't any deeper in trance than when he had started so, when he woke him up at the end of the session, he asked whether he had found the visualization difficult. 'Not at all,' said the patient. 'I could see the lift clearly. The problem was that by the time we got down to the ground floor, we had minus six people in there!'

All the images used in deepening must be soothing and relaxing. Obviously one could not use the lift technique for someone who suffered from claustrophobia, nor would it be sensible to ask a patient who suffered from hay fever to imagine taking a stroll through a garden in the height of summer. Sometimes the patient may be asked to pick his own visualization – whatever he finds relaxing, such as a walk by the sea or in the country, or lying on a beach in the hot sun. One of the most important things about this type of visualization is that the patient should be able to be by himself in his imagination. His beach, for example, should be a deserted one, not one on which people are packed like sardines. For children, however, it is sometimes helpful to let them imagine an adult with them – perhaps the therapist or a parent.

Sometimes the hypnotherapist may use a non-visual technique to deepen the trance. For example, he may count to ten, or to twenty, synchronizing the counting with the patient's breathing, and telling him that, as the count continues, so he will become more and more relaxed. Another method that uses the breathing is to ask the patient to take a very deep breath and hold it. He is then told to let it out very gradually and, as he does so, he will feel himself sinking down, deeper asleep. This can be repeated several times. Or the therapist may pick up the patient's arm, holding it loosely by the sleeve, and tell him that, when he drops the arm gently back into the patient's lap, it will be a signal to him to go deeper asleep.

The patient's arm is also used in a method called hand levitation. There are several variations of this, but in all of them the patient's arm lifts into the air, without the patient himself being aware of actively lifting it. In one form of the technique, the patient is asked to imagine a balloon, bobbing above his head. The string is tied to his wrist and he can feel it tugging it upwards. Gradually his arm lifts up, pulled by the balloon. Because the patient is already in a suggestible state, being in a light hypnotic trance, he will usually be able to picture and feel the balloon and his arm will start to rise. However, the more scientifically minded patient, aware that an air-filled balloon could not possibly tug his wrist upwards may not be able to visualize this. This is why some therapists may mention, in passing, that the balloon is filled with helium, a gas that is lighter than air! After the patient's hand has lifted, the therapist tells him that the string will be cut and his arm will fall back into his lap. As his hand touches his lap, this will be a signal for him to go deeper asleep. Because this method is a combination of visualization and the 'signal' technique, it may cause the patient to go into a deeper trance than either used alone.

One would think that the average doctor's surgery would be a most unsuitable place in which to practise hypnosis, with telephones ringing and people coming and going outside the door. But all these noises can be put to use and, far from detracting from the level of the trance, can actually add to it. This is achieved very simply by the therapist telling the patient, 'If, while you are in hypnosis, you hear any sounds other than my voice, you will take them as a signal to go even deeper asleep.'

Ego-Strengthening

Once the patient is as deep in trance as the therapist considers necessary, the treatment proper begins. Since most conditions which respond to hypnotherapy involve some degree of anxiety and self-doubt, the technique of ego-strengthening is widely used and forms an important part of the treatment for many patients. It consists of certain suggestions given by the therapist concerning the way the patient feels about himself. At a very basic level it may just consist of telling him that he will feel more confident and self-assured and will be able to cope better with his life. Or visualizations may be used. One that is very useful is to ask the patient to visualize a large round blob which is an ovum, or egg, with many, many sperm swimming towards it, looking like tadpoles. He is asked to identify with one sperm and to watch it as, swimming very strongly, it pulls ahead of the others and, reaching the egg first, fertilizes it. And, as it does so, he is asked to feel the sense of achievement that comes with winning a race. He is told that this is the way in which his life began, with a sperm fertilizing an egg. The very first event in his life was a triumph and therefore, having proved himself capable of success by winning that race, there is no reason why he should doubt his capabilities in other directions.

Another technique used for ego-strengthening is to ask the patient to remember some incident when he really felt pleased and satisfied with himself and to project himself back to it (often it is something that occurred in childhood, such as doing well at school or winning a competition). He is told that he will remember exactly how he felt on that occasion and will be able to relive his pride in achievement. Once he has done this, he is asked to do something physical, such as clenching his fist or rubbing his fingers together, and he is told that each time he performs that movement he will be able to recapture that same feeling of achievement and satisfaction. So, if at any time he is feeling low or unsure of himself, he will be able to use this technique in order to boost his self-confidence.

Some people, while being able to cope well with their normal routine, find that certain situations cause them to feel nervous or to lose confidence. Here visualization may be very helpful in enabling the patient to picture himself confronting such situations with assurance. For example, let us suppose that the patient is a man who holds a responsible position in a large organization. He enjoys his job and is good at it, but from time to time he has to give lectures which he dreads. Having to stand up and speak in public terrifies him but, because he doesn't have to do it very often, it hasn't affected the rest of his work. However, he is aware that, because of his fear, the standard of his lectures is poor, no matter how well he prepares them, and he always spends a miserable week in a state of nerves before each lecture. In a case such as this, the patient may first be asked to imagine himself going about his normal work and perhaps doing one particular thing extremely well and being congratulated by his superiors. This would be followed by a suggestion that, because he knows that he is very capable in his everyday work, this feeling of confidence will remain with him through the session of hypnotherapy. He is then asked to see himself going into the lecture room, with his notes in his hand. Gradually, he imagines himself giving the talk, still retaining the feeling of confidence. He notices how attentive the members of the audience are and how much they seem to be enjoying what he has to say. When he has finished, they all applaud enthusiastically, boosting his confidence still further.

The great advantage of visualizing a stressful situation under hypnosis, as opposed to experiencing the real thing, is that, should the patient start to feel nervous, the scene can be stopped immediately. His feeling of confidence is then built up once more before the visualization is re-started. Once the patient has pictured himself giving a lecture a number of times and has remained confident throughout, it will start to become easier for him to do so in real life. A technique like this would normally be used in conjunction with other forms of ego-strengthening.

After the ego-strengthening techniques, the rest of the session will usually be spent in dealing with any complaints that need more specific treatment. (Chapter Six deals with individual complaints and shows how they might be treated.) In addition, some other more general techniques may be taught. For example, the patient may be told that if, when he is in a stressful situation, he repeats a certain phrase to himself (such as 'calm and relaxed'), he will feel his anxieties and tensions disappear. Or he may be taught to imagine that he is surrounded by an invisible but protective barrier which he can put up at any time to prevent himself from being upset by other people or by situations. One version of this, which can be used by anyone, even without learning it under hypnosis, is to imagine oneself dressed in a long cloak made of dark blue velvet. It pulls in snugly round the neck, goes right down to the feet and overlaps in front, thus covering the whole body. Inside it is very roomy and is lined with a light silky material. The patient is told that within the cloak is his own inner space which cannot be invaded by anyone else. The cloak will protect him from violation by the 'outside world'.

Self-hypnosis

During the first session of hypnosis, or sometimes the second, the patient may be taught how to hypnotize himself. Self-hypnosis is a vital part of the treatment for many patients. Normally, they will only attend for a session with the therapist once a week or once a fortnight, and in between the sessions it is the self-hypnosis that keeps the treatment going. It's like the practice that one does between visits to the piano teacher – the more often one practises, the better one becomes. And so most patients will be asked to set aside about 20 minutes a day in which to put themselves into hypnosis. During this session they may practise the various relaxation techniques that they have learned, or they may use relaxing visualizations, such as imagining themselves walking in a garden or lying on a beach (the same visualizations that can be used as deepening techniques), or they may be given specific visualizations to use. For example, the man who was scared of lecturing might be asked to picture himself giving a lecture while remaining relaxed and comfortable.

There are two methods that the patient may use to put himself into hypnosis. Some practitioners like to make a recording of the session and give the cassette to the patient to listen to. In this way, his practice at home will be identical to his session with the therapist. Other practitioners give the patient a post-hypnotic suggestion that a certain series of words or phrases will have the effect of putting him into hypnosis when he repeats them to himself. This type of self-hypnosis is more flexible since it enables the patient to concentrate on whatever he thinks is most necessary on any particular occasion, and to make the session as long or as short as he wishes.

The patient is always given a series of unconnected words or two unconnected phrases with which to induce his trance, never a single word or single phrase which might come up in conversation and which might result in a susceptible subject going into hypnosis at an inappropriate moment. And, because it could be dangerous to go into hypnosis under certain conditions, other precautions must also be taken, whichever method the patient is going to use. These precautions take the form of suggestions given to the patient while he is still in hypnosis. He is told that, when attempting self-hypnosis, he will only go into a trance, having turned on the tape or repeated the 'formula', if it is safe for him to do so. (I know of one man who found self-hypnosis very easy and who, on one occasion, while having a long relaxing bath, decided to put himself into hypnosis – but couldn't because his subconscious mind knew that it wasn't safe to be hypnotized while lying in the bath.) Having been taught how to put himself into a trance, the patient will be told how to wake himself up. He will also be told that if anything happens while he is in hypnosis that needs his immediate attention, he will wake up straight away and be fully alert to deal with it. The emphasis here is on something that needs immediate attention, rather than just something happening to attract his attention. So, for example, if he smells burning he will automatically wake up, whereas if the telephone rings he can decide whether or not he wants to answer it.

These precautions are, of course, absolutely essential to the safety of the patient and their inclusion or omission by a therapist who teaches self-hypnosis will give a good idea as to whether or not he is qualified to practise. Hypnosis is a very easy technique to learn – anyone can put someone else into a hypnotic trance. Unfortunately, if one doesn't know what to do with it or how to control it, it can become a very dangerous technique, so it is vital that one should always go to a therapist who has had adequate training. Self-hypnosis is perfectly safe if one has been taught by a qualified therapist, since he will not allow the patient to do anything that might cause him harm. Many doctors and dentists who use hypnosis will, while the patient is still in a trance, tell him that he will not allow himself to be hypnotized by anyone other than a doctor or a dentist. Psychotherapists and other trained hypnotherapists will use a different form of words, but the intention is the same – to prevent the patient from being hypnotized by someone who has no knowledge of what might occur once the subject is in a trance and no training in how to deal with it.

Stage Hypnosis

It was the dangers inherent in the use of hypnosis that led to the passing of the Hypnotism Act by Parliament in 1952. Unfortunately, it still allows hypnosis to be used as a public entertainment, although regulating it more closely than before. Under the terms of the Act, an 'exhibition, demonstration or performance' of hypnotism can only be given if permitted by the local authority, which has the power to 'regulate or prohibit' such a performance. In addition, if a hypnotist uses a subject who is under the age of 18, he is liable to be fined.

However, none of the provisions of this Act would have protected Miss Diana Rains-Bath, who, in March 1952, only months before the Hypnotism Act was passed by Parliament, sued a stage hypnotist, Ralph Slater, at Sussex Assizes for negligence and assault. The details of this case show clearly the dangers that may be involved in the use of hypnotism as a form of entertainment, when the hypnotist has had no formal training and knows nothing about his subjects.

Miss Rains-Bath had attended a performance given by Slater at the Brighton Hippodrome in 1948, when she was 19 years old, and, together with a friend, had volunteered to be a subject. Of the 15 or 20 people who went up on stage, she was one of three who were picked out, after tests of hypnotic susceptibility, to be used in the demonstration. She was obviously a naturally deep subject and, once Slater had hypnotized her, he apparently told her, 'You will do just what I tell you.' He then went over to one of the other subjects and Miss Rains-Bath woke herself up. However, Slater came back to her and forced her head forward, commanding her to sleep. She was aware at the time that this manoeuvre was painful and it was upon this that the assault charge was based.

When she was again in a trance, Slater told her that her chair was getting hot and, as a result, she jumped up. He also told her that, after she woke up, if he stamped on the floor, she would get up from her seat and shout 'Peanuts', something that she later did, when she was back in the audience. This was all fairly harmless stuff and the sort of thing to which someone who had volunteered to be a subject would put up no defence. However, Slater then told Miss Rains-Bath that she was going to be like a little baby that is frightened and crying for its mother. And, indeed, she did start crying and calling out, 'Mummy, Mummy!' Again, this was not a suggestion that actually threatened her or went against her moral principles and therefore it is not surprising that, being a good subject, she complied with it. As the expert medical witness who was called in court remarked, it would have been a different matter if she had been told to take her clothes off. However, the fact that she tried to wake herself up at the beginning of the act suggests that her subconscious mind wasn't altogether happy about doing 'just what she was told'.

All might still have been well, but for the fact that Slater did not remove the suggestion of feeling frightened and wanting her mother before waking her up. When Miss Rains-Bath awoke, she felt, so she said, tired and dazed. However, this passed and for a week or so she felt her normal happy self. But then, one morning, she woke feeling very frightened. She started to feel depressed and weepy and lost interest in everything. She told the court, 'My mind seemed miles away and I could not concentrate on anything.' The depression lifted but then returned and this became a regular cycle so that she started to have periods of depression lasting a week or more. Gradually the periods during which she was depressed became longer until she was happy only occasionally. She consulted several doctors and, finally, was seen by hypnotherapist Dr S. J. Van Pelt, who at that time was President of the British Society of Medical Hypnosis. He treated her over a period of four months in 1950 and, finally, after 23 sessions of hypnotherapy, the depression was cured.

It should be noted that Miss Rains-Bath's friend, who was also hypnotized and told to cry for her mother, felt 'rather peculiar' after leaving the theatre but had no long-lasting effects. There could have been several reasons for this – she may have been a less susceptible subject, she may have been a generally less emotional person, or Slater may have remembered to remove the suggestion before he woke her up.

In court, Miss Rains-Bath's counsel, Mr John Flowers, QC, questioned Dr Van Pelt about the treatment he had given her. He asked whether it would have been likely to have succeeded if it had not been hypnosis that had caused the problem. 'No,' replied Dr Van Pelt. And was it dangerous to tell a hypnotized girl that she would feel frightened and cry for her mummy? 'It is a foolish thing to tell anybody because crying brings along with it deep fundamental emotions which have a great effect on the mind and such suggestion could cause much harm.' Dr Van Pelt agreed with Mr Flowers that the suggestion should have been removed before the subject woke and that the manoeuvre employed by Slater in which he forced the girl's neck forward could have been dangerous, since it interfered with the circulation and the blood pressure.

In his defence, Slater told the court how he had become a hypnotist. As a boy he 'did not do too well at other subjects' and became interested in psychology. From this, he developed an interest in hypnotism. 'I found there was only one way to learn hypnotism, which was to study and practise.' (A qualified hypnotherapist would disagree strongly with this – book-learning is no way to learn hypnosis, nor is practising on subjects without supervision.) Slater said that he had practised hypnotism for many years in America (although he was, in fact, British) and had been giving public demonstrations for over 15 years. He had, he said, hypnotized well over 25,000 people, had used 'mass hypnotism by radio' and had 'never had any claim against me as a result of hypnotic demonstrations'. In this he was surely fortunate, since with mass hypnotism he could have had no idea at all of who might have been listening to him. Indeed, Mr Flowers mentioned that, in a book written by Slater, he had said that hysterical people should not be hypnotized – but how, asked Mr

Flowers, could he know whether 20 strangers coming up onto a stage had hysterical temperaments?

The jury was in no doubt that it was the hypnotist who had caused Miss Rains-Bath's condition and found him guilty (although this verdict was later overturned by the Appeal Court on a point of law). They had been warned by the judge that they were to decide only whether Slater had been guilty of negligence and assault, not whether it was desirable that hypnotism should be allowed to be practised as a public entertainment. The fact that it was necessary for him to mention this makes it clear that, in some minds at least, there was a very strong doubt as to the desirability of using hypnosis in this way.

Since the Hypnotism Act did nothing to outlaw such entertainments, the public use of hypnosis still causes concern among qualified hypnotherapists. This is not due to any form of professional jealousy, but is entirely concerned with the possible use of unsuitable subjects and the lack of safeguards for the demonstration. There are certain people who are unsuitable to be hypnotized, such as those suffering from depression or other forms of mental illness. And there are those, like Miss Rains-Bath, who are particularly susceptible to certain suggestions affecting the emotions. As is evident from her case, although the stage hypnotist has methods for picking out subjects susceptible to hypnosis, he has no way of knowing whether their mental state is suitable. In addition, the lack of safeguards may result in some post-hypnotic suggestion being still in force when the subject leaves the theatre, which may, as we have seen, cause that person considerable distress.

However, in 1977, as a result of lobbying by Dr David Waxman (later to be President of the British Society of Medical and Dental Hypnosis), the Home Office asked the newly formed Federation of Stage Hypnotists to consider devising a code of practice. Representatives of the Federation met Dr Waxman and two other members of the BSMDH, and a code was worked out. According to this, members of the Federation would not attempt to carry out any form of therapy on stage, would not perform age regression and would not suggest anything improper to a subject nor give him any substance (to take or smell) that might harm him. They would not suggest to a subject that he was going rigid. (This was a favourite of some hypnotists, who would make the subject lie with just his head and his heels supported by chairs and then apply a heavy weight to his body to show that he was 'like a board'.) And finally, all post-hypnotic suggestions were to be removed before the end of each performance.

This was a considerable step forward – such a code of conduct would certainly have protected Miss Rains-Bath. Unfortunately, the code is voluntary and not all stage hypnotists belong to the Federation. Indeed, I recently saw a poster advertising a hypnotist's act in which it was promised that he would treat members of the audience in order to stop them from smoking. And at the bottom of the poster was printed in large letters, 'THE SHOW THE DOCTORS TRIED TO BAN'.

CHAPTER FIVE

REGRESSION

Perhaps the technique that causes the most disagreement between hypnotherapists is that of regression. Some are vigorously in favour of its use, while others are just as vigorously against it. Some are happy to use so-called 'age regression', in which the patient is taken back to early periods in his life, while others will go further and regress the patient to the time when he was a foetus lying in his mother's womb, or a baby in the process of being born. Still others, probably the minority, do 'past life regression' in which patients are taken back in time and are encouraged to relive events that supposedly happened to them in previous lives. Obviously, to those who do not believe in reincarnation, past life regression is a nonsense and the stories that the patients tell while in hypnosis pure fabrication, based on things that they have seen and read.

It is, of course, possible to fabricate under hypnosis. The visualizations in which a patient sees himself coping calmly with something that has frightened him in the past are all a form of make-believe. So too are the techniques used to deepen the hypnotic trance, although these are not true fabrications, for when the patient wakes up he is aware that he was not really wandering in a garden or going down in a lift. But the whole object of the ego-strengthening type of visualization is to persuade the patient's subconscious mind that what he is imagining is real.

The fact that hypnotized subjects seem able to remember things about their childhood which have long been forgotten, or even repressed, suggests that the memory can be greatly improved while in hypnosis. However, Professor

Martin Orne, past President of the International Society of Hypnosis, once observed in a lecture that it seemed very strange that the Almighty should provide each of us with a sort of mental tape recorder which recorded all the events of our lives but which could only be turned on by a hypnotist! And, as Professor Orne has shown in some experiments, the 'memories' that the patients produce, even of recent events, can be far from the actual truth.

Hypnosis has been used quite widely in the United States to assist in the interrogation of witnesses to crimes, in an attempt to enable them to recall more about the event than they otherwise might. However, in certain states, such as California, Arizona and Pennsylvania, the State Supreme Courts have ruled that information given by a witness under hypnosis is no longer admissible in a court of law. A number of investigators have performed experiments to try to see what the exact effect of hypnosis is upon a witness. One thing that most experiments demonstrate is that those witnesses who have recalled additional information while under hypnosis are likely, afterwards, to be very certain of the truth of what they have remembered. Thus it seems that one of the effects of hypnosis is to persuade the subject that his memory is accurate – even if it isn't. In addition, it is perfectly possible for a subject to tell lies under hypnosis, so that the fact that he gave certain information while in hypnosis is not even a guarantee that he thought that what he was saying was the truth. Several investigators have noted the tendency of witnesses to confabulate while in hypnosis – in other words, if they come to a gap in their memory, they unconsciously make something up to fill it – and then later come to believe that this made-up information is true.

Professor Martin Orne, who has done a great deal of work on forensic hypnosis (that is, the use of hypnosis in criminal cases), has shown that it is perfectly possible to put something into the mind of a hypnotized subject that he will later state to be the truth. And this needn't be the result of an unscrupulous hypnotist 'nobbling' the witnesses – it could be done in all innocence, simply by using a phrase or sentence that might suggest something to the patient's subconscious mind. In a programme on hypnosis shown on BBC television in 1982, Professor Orne hypnotized a subject who had said, before the session, that on a certain night during the week she had slept soundly and had not woken once. He showed how very easy it was to use what in legal terms might be called leading questions to persuade the patient that she had, in fact, been woken up during that night by a bang in the street outside. The experiment was so successful that when the patient awoke from hypnosis she was firmly convinced, not only that she had been woken by a bang on that particular night, but that it had taken her some time to get to sleep again.

However, although it is possible to demonstrate that such 'memories' can be fabricated, it does not necessarily mean that all memories produced under hypnosis are false. In fact, most of us have our own experience of hypnosis helping to jog the memory. We have probably all at some time forgotten a name or an important fact – something we couldn't look up and that kept nagging at us during the course of the day, without anything coming to mind. And then, at night, just as we were dropping off to sleep, we suddenly opened our eyes and said the name or fact that had eluded us all day. The state between sleeping and waking, although fairly fleeting, is very similar to a hypnotic trance, and it is as we drift into this state of relaxation that the memory that we are seeking comes rushing back.

There are certainly cases of people being put into hypnosis and remembering things far back in their childhood with an accuracy which is later confirmed by parents or other members of the family. There are also cases of people 'remembering' events that apparently never happened to them. So does it matter whether the event is real or imagined? If one is talking in terms of hypnotherapy and not the forensic use of hypnosis, the answer is probably no. The object of regression therapy is to bring out something from the patient's subconscious mind which is troubling him. For example, a patient may be suffering from claustrophobia as a result of having been accidentally locked in a cupboard when he was three years old. His conscious mind has probably long since forgotten the incident, knowing that the episode was a long time ago and no longer relevant to his life today. But the emotions associated with the experience are still active in his subconscious mind and, whenever he is in a confined space, he is subconsciously reminded of the emotions evoked by being shut in a cupboard. As a result he starts to feel apprehension and fear. If the original event that caused the present symptoms was particularly traumatic, then it is possible for the conscious mind to blot it out completely. But it is not possible for the subconscious mind to blot out the associated emotions, and it is from these that the problem stems.

It has been found that to bring out into the open the events that precipitated conditions such as claustrophobia may help the patient considerably in dealing with the problem. Many of us know that feeling of being anxious but not knowing what is causing the anxiety. Then, suddenly, we will become aware of what it is that is nagging and, just as suddenly, with that realization, the anxiety becomes greatly reduced and falls into perspective. The very fact of not knowing the cause was, in itself, contributing to the anxiety. Similarly, anxiety or emotions related to past events that we do not remember are very often out of all perspective to the causative event. For the patient to be able to remember and talk about the cause and see it as it relates to his life today is often a major step towards his recovery.

But what of 'memories' brought up by the patient under hypnosis that appear to have no basis in truth? Can they be of any use? Here again, the answer seems to be yes. There are many cases in which patients have been helped by visualizing and talking about some traumatic event which appears never to have happened. Remembering a genuine past event can allay the anxiety associated with it by focusing the attention on the cause of that anxiety. But an apparently imagined focus appears to act in the same way. In other words, it seems not to matter whether the 'memory' is genuine or imagined, because in either case it seems to bring something out of the patient's subconscious mind which either is, or symbolizes, the cause of his anxieties, and it can therefore act to bring these anxieties into perspective.

Between the two fields of regression to a younger age and regression to a past life lies regression to the time when the patient was in his mother's womb and when he was born. One might wonder why regression to this period should have any relevance to a patient's problems but, according to practitioners of 'primal therapy', the brainchild of Dr Arthur Janov, an American psychologist, the events occurring before, during and after birth can, if traumatic, affect the patient's emotional state for the rest of his life. The basic theory behind primal therapy is that unmet needs occurring early in life cause physical or psychological pain. If the pain is very severe and, because of its severity, it is suppressed, it cannot be lost from the system. Suppressed pain may be converted into tension and this, in turn, may produce other symptoms. However, if the patient switches off his awareness of the tension or of the pain, psychotic mental states may occur in which the patient loses touch with reality. The tension felt by a patient who is suffering from a neurosis is used by him as a protective mechanism, for if he allowed himself to relax, he would be able to feel the pain which his body and mind are suppressing. Primal therapy consists of allowing the patient to feel and deal with the pain from which he is suffering, in order to relieve him of his neurosis.

Birth is a fairly traumatic business and, if the primal therapists are to be believed, it is small wonder that so many people have difficulty in coping with life without anxiety and tension. Ideally, a child should be wanted from the start, delivered normally and easily, and held and loved by its mother from the moment the cord is cut. However, often this is not possible. Despite modern obstetric methods, some births are still difficult and a certain percentage of deliveries are by forceps or Caesarean section. And sometimes babies have to be whisked away from their mothers immediately after birth, either because they are premature or sickly or because the mother is unwell.

A child who is unable to grow properly in the womb because of an inadequate dietary intake by his mother, or because she smokes or drinks heavily, is going to have unmet needs which, in primal terms, equal pain. Birth itself is bound to cause pain, say the primal therapists, because, after nine months of comfort and warmth and safety in the womb, suddenly the child is being turned out to face something quite unknown. The passage down the birth canal can be very frightening and, if it takes a long time, may cause claustrophobia in later life. If there are difficulties with the delivery because the baby has the umbilical cord round his neck, this, too, may be associated with difficulties later in life such as anorexia, speech problems or problems with breathing (such as asthma). And if the child, after going through all this trauma, does not have the immediate comfort and warmth of the mother's love and is not able to suckle, other problems may develop owing to the tension precipitated by unmet needs.

It can be seen, therefore, that in the treatment of patients whose problems date back to traumas experienced around the time of birth, regression under hypnosis can be extremely useful. The technique is to allow the patient to relive and experience fully the pain that he felt at the time in order to get it out of his system, and to enable him to see that it is no longer appropriate to his life today.

Many phobias appear to have their origins in a traumatic event and sometimes this is remembered consciously – for example someone with a fear of dogs may remember being frightened by a dog when he was a small child. In this case, it is not necessary to get the patient to remember the incident – he already does – but it is the recognition of the inappropriateness of his emotions to his present state which is important. At the age of four or five a dog may seem enormous, whereas to an adult it is just a small animal. And it is possible to accomplish this change of thinking by suggestions given under hypnosis.

Very often, the therapist may ask the patient to go back in his mind to the incident (or one of the incidents) which precipitated his present problem. He may start to describe an incident in his childhood or around the time of his birth, or he may, as psychologist Dr Edith Fiore found, start to describe a 'past life'. Dr Fiore, who says in her book *You Have Been Here Before* (Sphere, 1980) that she is neither a staunch believer nor a non-believer in reincarnation, had been treating patients using age regression under hypnosis. One day a young man with severe sexual problems came to see her and she asked him, under hypnosis, to go back to the origin of his problems. His reply was, 'Two or three lifetimes ago, I was a Catholic priest.' Knowing that this patient believed in reincarnation, she felt after the session that his colourful and emotional description of life as a seventeenth-century Italian priest was a fantasy. However, the next time he came to see her, his sexual problems had resolved. As a result, she started to use the technique of past life regression on other patients, often with extremely good results. As she says in her book, whether the images and stories that are conjured up are reality or fantasy doesn't matter, as long as they get results.

Of course, past life regression is not always done with therapy in mind. Sometimes it is done on an experimental basis to see whether or not reincarnation can be 'proved'. An early case of supposed past life regression, that of 'Bridey Murphy', caused quite a sensation in the mid-1950s and a book on the subject, *The Search for Bridey Murphy* by Morey Bernstein, was published by Hutchinson in 1956. The subject had apparently regressed to the last century and taken on the persona of a young Irish girl. However, after the intitial amazement, further research into the subject's background suggested that she knew – or had known – a considerable amount about the time and places she described, and that the regression could therefore very easily be a fabrication based on her knowledge. It is only when it seems impossible that subjects could have known the facts that they produce during regression, and when these facts are verifiable, that it is possible to suggest that the case may truly be one of past life regression.

My first introduction to this fascinating field was when, some years ago, I heard a tape recording made by a hypnotist in which he regressed a young woman back to the reign of George III. In this regression she became a young man – a gipsy – and spoke with a smattering of Romany words. She was able to give her name and she described how she and her cousin were in a town where a fair was being held. When a storm started, the two men took shelter in a barn which was then struck by lightning and both were killed. The young woman, said the hypnotist, had never been to this town. However, when taken there after she had described it in her regression, she recognized the older parts – and found a tombstone with the gipsy's name on it in the graveyard. Of course, it is impossible to say whether or not she had really ever been there – it is impossible to remember every single place that one has ever visited. And I am unsure whether the 'Romany' she spoke was ever verified. But it was a fascinating story.

The first introduction that many people had to the idea of past life regression was through the television programme and book *More Lives Than One?* (Pan, 1976), in which Jeffrey Iverson investigated the work of Arnall Bloxham, President of the British Society of Hypnotherapists, who had achieved considerable recognition in Cardiff, where he was then practising. Iverson, a producer with the BBC, had thought that Bloxham would make an interesting subject for a television programme and began his research by listening to recordings that Bloxham had made of hundreds of hours of regressions. To his surprise, he found that most of these subjects told stories of very ordinary, boring lives. As he wrote in the book, 'If what the psychiatrists said was true, and people were fantasizing about themselves, then most were pitching their fantasies modestly and surprisingly low.' But Iverson was not content with just listening to tapes – he wanted to see regression in action. At the start of his research for the programme, he watched Bloxham hypnotize a colleague and regress her to a life in ancient Greece (a period in which she had apparently no interest at all). He found this most impressive, particularly as it was clear that Bloxham did not direct the regression in any way and asked no leading questions.

Among the tapes Iverson found several regressions which were particularly interesting and which were all produced by the same subject, referred to in his book as 'Jane'. She was therefore invited to undergo further sessions which were filmed for the programme. In all, she regressed to six separate 'lives', of which three were particularly fascinating.

In the first she was Livonia, the wife of a tutor of Latin and Greek, living on the outskirts of York in the third century. In another, which is the one that most people who saw the programme seem to remember, she was Rebecca, a Jewish woman who was a victim of the York massacre in 1190. And in the third, and perhaps the most interesting, she was Alison, a serving girl to a nobleman in the Loire valley in the fifteenth century. Coming from the same part of Wales, Jeffrey Iverson found that he had been to the same school as Jane and was able to ascertain quite easily that the periods of history involved in these regressions had not been on the school syllabus. Furthermore, Jane said that she had never been to the Loire valley nor studied its history. And yet she was able to describe the house in which she had lived as a servant (which still stands) and to talk, correctly, about the relationships of various people at Court. She was also able to talk about the artists who had painted and sculpted the works owned by her master. Here her knowledge seemed truly remarkable, since one of the artists appeared only to be mentioned in specialist textbooks. But perhaps the most exciting part was when she described a 'golden apple' prized by her master; after much research, a list of items that he had owned was found by a French historian and in that list was a 'grenade [or pomegranate] of gold' – in other words, an item of gold that looked very much like an apple.

Past life regression was the subject of another television programme shown on Channel Four in 1985 which followed through an experiment carried out by Australian hypnotherapist Peter Ramster. Out of the many patients he had regressed he picked four woman who not only produced vivid and detailed descriptions of their past lives but, in addition, had never visited the countries in which they said they had lived (England, Scotland, France and Germany); indeed, one of them had never been out of Australia. All the regression was done in Australia and as much information as possible was requested from the subjects and recorded. Then the four women were taken to Europe, to the places to which they had apparently regressed, and were asked to find their way around.

One of the four, who had described life as a Jewish girl in Nazi Germany, found that the streets were not as she had described them, nor were buildings in the places that she had said they were. However, the woman who described her life in a grand house in France was able to take Peter Ramster on a guided tour of that house (now derelict). She had also described (accurately, as it turned out) a house, several miles away, at which she had spent a number of summers and, without looking at a map, she was able to give directions which took them from one house to the other. When the woman who had regressed to a small English village in the eighteenth century had been in hypnosis, she had talked about a friend of hers whose cottage had a strange pattern carved in the stone floor. Before leaving Australia, she was asked to draw that pattern. When she arrived in the village, the cottage still stood, although it had for many years been used as a hen-house. But when the hens were turned out and the floor cleaned, there was the pattern on the floor. And, equally amazing was the woman who had described her life as a doctor in a Scottish town and who was able to point out where the Seamen's Mission had stood in the early nineteenth century (a fact unknown to local historians, who were only able to confirm it after delving into records). And finding, without difficulty, the building which had once been the medical school, she told the archivist what several of the rooms had been used for and where the gentlemen's toilet had been – facts that were verified by looking at a map which was kept in the University archives but which had apparently never been reproduced elsewhere.

Although such results are greeted with delight by those

who believe in reincarnation, there are, of course, people who feel that there must be some other explanation. One of the arguments often put forward by those who feel that past life regressions must be imaginary concerns language. If someone spoke Romany, or French, or Italian, or ancient Egyptian in a previous life and if, in hypnosis, they appear to be reliving their experiences in that life, then one would expect them to recount those experiences in the language that they spoke at the time. This would seem to be a very sound argument. Some subjects, however, do speak partly in their 'previous' language (such as the 'gipsy' with his smattering of Romany) and partly in their present-day language. Others will speak only in their present language but will offer words in their previous tongue if requested. Some appear unable to recall any of their previous language although remembering quite a lot about the relevant lifetime. One way in which such phenomena may be explained is this: it is rather like the situation of someone who, as a small child, was brought up in a household in which French was spoken fluently. At the age of five, he was taken away and put in another household where only English was spoken, and he never spoke French again. At the age of 65 he is asked, in English, about his life as a small child: he may be able to remember certain events quite vividly, but he will describe them in English. However, if there were certain words or phrases that made a particular impression on him (perhaps a term of endearment used towards him), he is likely to repeat that in the original French. When pressed, he may even be able to remember some other French words that have remained dormant in his mind for 60 years.

Similarly, when people describe, in hypnosis, what it was like to be born, they do so in adult terms, although obviously they knew no language at all at the time. On one occasion, a colleague of mine asked a patient to go back in time to the first incident which had contributed to his present problems. Knowing something of the patient's childhood, he expected this to be an event when he was about four or five years old and was therefore rather surprised when he was told, 'I'm lying near a naked woman.' The patient went on, 'There are other people about. And I've got a rushing noise in my ears. There's a strong artificial light and I can hear bells. I'm hot and I feel tingling and unpleasant. I feel as though I'm floating – it seems as though I'm being lifted up. And now I'm shouting. I feel very frustrated – I want something but I don't know what it is.' He was, of course, describing events shortly after he had been born. And although, as a newborn baby, he could only express his frustration by crying (or 'shouting'), he was now describing it in the language of a 30 year-old man.

There are many methods that are used to get patients to regress. The simplest is that used by Arnall Bloxham in which the patient is just asked to go back in time. Dr Edith Fiore's method is to suggest to the patient that he travel back through time and space while she counts slowly to ten; when she reaches ten, while still being himself, the patient will find that he is in another time and another place and another body, but all of these will be relevant to his present problems. A method which is useful when one is regressing a patient only a short distance, perhaps a matter of a few months or years, is to ask him to imagine a calendar and see it going backwards until the required date is reached.

It is necessary for a patient to be able to go into a medium-depth or deep trance in order to be regressed, and even then there may be resistance, particularly if he has been suppressing a painful memory for years. There are ways to get round this, however. One method is for the therapist to say that he is going to count to five, and that while he is doing so something will come into the patient's mind that will give a clue to the cause of his problems. This 'something' may be something he sees, such as a scene or a face, or a non-visual clue such as a noise or a snatch of tune, a smell, or even an emotion. The patient is told to allow his mind to go completely blank and just allow whatever it is to come into his mind; it may appear to have no relevance to the problem and so he is not to discard any thought or emotion that suddenly appears, however trivial it may seem. This technique needs a reasonable depth of trance, because it is important that the conscious mind is overridden by the subconscious. A patient whose trance is too light will either come up with what he consciously thinks is relevant or will come up with nothing, saying, 'I'm sorry, I really can't think of anything that might have caused it.'

A similar method is to ask the hypnotized patient to give three letters of the alphabet off the top of his head. Then he is asked, again without thinking about it, to say three words, each beginning with one of the letters, and each of which will be relevant to his problem. And finally, he is asked to put each of the words into a sentence. With both this method and the previous one, what has come into the patient's mind or the sentences he produces have then to be developed and enlarged upon. Of course, using these methods the patient may not regress, since there may be things in his life as it is at present that are of great relevence to his problem, and it may be these that come to mind.

Often patients are nervous that there may be something traumatic in their past which they are going to be required to remember. However, although it is often important to re-experience the emotions associated with traumatic events, in order to get them out of the system, the edge can be taken off by suggestions from the therapist that the patient will remain calm and relaxed throughout the session. In some way the patient can experience the emotion in the previous period, while at the same time remaining relaxed in the present, and he is aware of being both in a different time and in the hypnotherapist's chair. Perhaps the closest analogy that one can get is that of watching a 'weepy' film on television. While dabbing at one's eyes with a handkerchief because of the moving events on the screen, one is still very much aware that the emotion one is feeling is relevant only to that film and not to one's life.

The image of the television set or the cinema screen can, in fact, be used to protect the patient from events that are very traumatic. Instead of being asked to go back and experience such events, he is asked to imagine that he is watching a film of them. He will be aware of the emotions that the person on the screen is going through because he is that person but, because he is detached from the scene, he will not be unduly upset by them. It is often helpful to take the patient on some time after the event to a more peaceful episode in order to show him that he survived the trauma and thus give him confidence in his own strength and resistance. Even in patients who see themselves dying in former lives, continuing on after the death will often produce a sense of peace and relaxation and, if they move forward into the current life, will show them that everything can be overcome. In *More Lives than One?* Jeffrey Iverson describes a patient of Arnall Bloxham's who was afraid of going to sleep in case he should die. Bloxham's solution was to regress the patient to previous lives and convince him that he had lived – and died – before and that therefore death should hold no surprises or terrors for him.

Another method of creating a sense of detachment from traumatic events, and one which is extremely useful when one is exploring the patient's current life from an early age, is the visualization of a 'Book of Life'. The patient is asked to imagine a bookshelf on which are several books labelled 'My Life: Volume 1', 'My Life: Volume 2', and so on, the number of volumes depending on the age of the patient. At the first session, he is asked to imagine himself taking down the first book, sitting down and opening it on his lap. Each page is like a television screen with a moving picture, and shows an event that is of significance in his life. Volume One will start with events when he was very young (perhaps up to the age of five or the time at which he started school). He is asked to look at each picture in turn and describe what is happening and how he feels about it. When he has talked at length about each picture and the emotions with which he associates it, he is given a choice. If he considers that the memories that the page conjured up were pleasant and happy ones, and he wants to keep them, then all he has to do is to turn the page over and go on to the next. If, however, the memories are unhappy or traumatic ones, then he can tear the page out, screw it up and throw it away – and it will never trouble him again. This is a particularly useful method when a series of minor events have contributed to a patient's problems, but less so when one or more very traumatic episodes are involved.

Obviously it is important that sessions of regression should not be too traumatic for the patient. Long-standing problems may take a number of sessions of hypnotherapy before they start to resolve and if the patient is going to be too scared to return for another session, then the technique is pointless. On some occasions, therefore, it may be necessary for the patient to be allowed to forget what has happened under hypnosis, while his subconscious mind works it out. Many hypnotherapists will routinely tell patients that when they wake up they will remember only the parts of the session with which the conscious mind is able to cope. The patient himself then has the choice as to what he remembers and what he forgets.

CHAPTER SIX

SOME COMMON CONDITIONS

AND THEIR TREATMENT

Hypnotherapy may be of value in the treatment of a wide variety of complaints. In this chapter, I shall discuss how a therapist might treat some of the conditions that he commonly sees. However, new methods of treatment are being developed all the time and many more exist than can be described in a single chapter. Therefore, a patient who goes to a hypnotherapist will not necessarily be treated with any of the methods mentioned here. Each therapist uses the techniques that seem to him to give the best results and the fact that two practitioners may use quite different methods does not mean that one is more skilled, or even more up to date, than the other. However, it may mean that sometimes a patient will get on better with one therapist than with another. This is something that hypnotherapists themselves recognize and is the reason why, occasionally, a patient may be referred from one to another.

Smoking

When hypnotherapy is mentioned, the first thing that most people think of is that it is an aid to stopping smoking. However, as I mentioned earlier on, it can only help patients who really want to give up. It may be of great value for those people who smoke purely from habit, but less beneficial for those who really enjoy the taste of the cigarette and get satisfaction from the ritual involved in smoking. However, if a patient enjoys smoking but also has a very strong reason to stop (such as a heart condition), hypnotherapy may still be of use, because the way that it works is to strengthen his resolve and will-power to do what he knows he must.

Many people who smoke do so as an aid to relaxation. If they become anxious or they are working under pressure, they find that smoking a cigarette will relieve the tension. However, hypnosis is a far better relaxation technique and if it can be used to teach the patient to relax, he should no longer need any artificial aids. While he is in a trance, the therapist may tell him that each day he will become more and more relaxed in his everyday life and will find that the situations that used to make him tense and anxious will no longer do so. And, as a result, he will no longer need to smoke because he will no longer feel the stress that the cigarettes used to relieve. Smoking was just a crutch – now he can rely on himself. This, of course, is a form of ego-strengthening, giving the patient confidence in his own abilities.

There are two courses that may be taken by people who plan to give up smoking, whether or not they are having hypnotherapy to help them. Some decide that on a certain day they will stop and not smoke again. Others like to cut down gradually until, finally, they stop. The choice of tactics depends very much on the individual patient. Some find one method a great deal easier than the other and, if a patient has a particular preference, it is as well for him to mention this to the hypnotherapist at the first session, so that the suggestions given will be appropriate to the intended course of action.

If a patient decides to give up gradually, he may be asked to record his progress on a chart and, while he is in hypnosis, he may be asked to visualize the chart as it will appear in two or three weeks' time, when he has cut down his smoking even further. He may also be asked to look ahead and see what the date will be when he finally gives up. If he has difficulty in seeing this date, it suggests that he is not too anxious to stop smoking and may well find it hard to do so. However, if he can see the date, he can be asked to imagine the events on the day on which he stops – the feeling of achievement and the delight of his family or workmates (whoever is currently complaining most about his smoking). These visualizations can be used by the patient when he practises his self-hypnosis and will re-inforce the work done at the sessions with the hypno-therapist. The encouragement of the patient's family in his efforts to give up is very important. It is very much harder to stop smoking when other members of the family continue to puff away regardless. The therapist may therefore encourage couples who smoke to give up to-gether.

Giving up smoking is not always easy even if one has the will-power to do it. Many patients, whether they give up suddenly or gradually, suffer from withdrawal effects, sometimes for a considerable period of time. Fortunately, since these are common, the therapist knows what form they are likely to take and can therefore give the patient post-hypnotic suggestions to stop or reduce them. The commonest effects that patients complain of are craving for a cigarette, irritability, insomnia and wanting to eat all the time. These are all things that may be treated – the irrita-bility and insomnia can be overcome simply by teaching the patient to relax. The therapist will usually have asked the patient when it is that he feels the greatest need for a cigar-ette – such as after a meal, with a cup of coffee or when on the telephone – and will give him specific suggestions that he will not feel any need at all to smoke at these times, or, or course, at any other. In order to help him to deal with these particularly difficult times, the patient may be given a special technique to use – for example, he may be told that, when the craving starts, he is to snap his fingers and immediately it will disappear and be replaced by a sensation of relaxation and well-being. And, to prevent the patient from eating excessively, he may be told that, although he may enjoy his food more, having given up smoking, he will not have any desire to eat more than he normally does.

Patients may find that they can do without cigarettes quite happily until they get into an environment where other people are smoking. Then, the smell of the smoke tempts them to accept any offer of a cigarette that is made. An important suggestion, therefore, is to tell the patient that, far from making him want to smoke, the smell of other people smoking will seem very unpleasant. Indeed, it will make him wonder why he ever smoked. Similarly, he may be told that if he does light a cigarette it will taste dreadful and he will put it out straight away. This is a very effective suggestion with some patients, who report a dramatic change in the flavour of tobacco.

Those suggestions which depend upon the subject experiencing something which, in fact, is not so may be more easily accepted by the subconscious mind if they are coupled with suggestions that are based on reality. For example, the patient may be told that when he stops smoking cigarettes he will find that his food will taste much better and that he will be able to smell pleasant smells far more readily. This, of course, would happen anyway, since the senses of taste and smell, which are subdued by smoking, will gradually return when the patient gives up. However, the very fact that it does happen, just as the hypnotherapist has told him, will encourage the patient's subconscious mind to believe everything else that he has been told under hypnosis. Thus, he may be told that it is because of his improved sense of taste that any cigarette he lights will taste so dreadful.

Patients may also be given 'automatic reaction' suggestions, such as, 'If someone offers you a cigarette, you will automatically say, "No thank you, I've given up."' In a good subject who is well motivated, this can be a very effective technique, since the reaction will occur without the patient even thinking about it and will therefore help him to avoid being tempted to have 'just one'. The technique is the same as that used when it was suggested to Miss Raines-Bath that she shout 'Peanuts' whenever the hypnotist stamped on the floor, as described in Chapter Four. What is a source of amusement in the hands of a stage hypnotist may be a very valuable therapeutic tool in the hands of a hypnotherapist.

Self-hypnosis is very important in the treatment of those who wish to give up smoking. The patient who practises it regularly seems to do far better than the one who doesn't. It may be, of course, that the patient who practises is more determined to succeed, but there is no doubt that his task is made easier by his increased ability to relax, greater self-reliance, and improved confidence in his own ability to stop smoking – all results of regular practice. Perhaps the best self-hypnosis schedule for a smoker is 20 minutes a day while he is in the process of giving up and until he feels that he is unlikely to relapse, followed by 20 minutes two or three times a week for the rest of his life. In this way, if he ever finds himself open to the temptation to start again, he will have the technique at hand to help him to resist.

Reaction to treatment varies considerably with individual patients. Some find no difficulty at all in stopping smoking or in cutting down and then stopping. Others take longer than they intended, but still finally give up. Others seem to get nowhere. If a patient has made no progress after three sessions of hypnosis, the likelihood of it being of help is small and he would probably be best advised to try another method (such as an acupuncture stud) or to return to hypnosis at a later date when he is feeling more positive about giving up smoking.

Some patients who have given up smoking, having had hypnotherapy, will start again, sometimes several years later. So a therapist may see people whom he treated several years earlier coming back, rather shame-faced, for a repeat performance. Usually they have let their practice of self-hypnosis lapse. Often they are worried about whether the therapy will work a second time. In most cases it does, although sometimes it may be harder to give up than on the previous occasion, the patient having lost faith in himself and his ability to control his habits. However, as with first-time patients, it is the motivation that is important, and patients who really want to give up will do so.

Insomnia

Insomnia is a common symptom and often occurs together with other more major conditions, such as anxiety or chronic pain. In such cases, one would expect the insomnia to resolve as the main cause of the patient's problems improved. However, it may also occur by itself, for no apparent reason, and in these cases hypnotherapy may prove useful.

It is essential, first of all, to take a very full history of the problem. It may appear to the patient that there is no reason why his sleep patterns have suddenly become disturbed, but a trained therapist may be able to see a very obvious reason and, naturally, in such a case the therapy would concentrate on the relief of the cause of the insomnia. For example, there are some people who don't allow anything to worry them. No matter what happens, they continue to show a cheerful face and carry on regardless. It's not that things *don't* worry them, it's just that they suppress such things and refuse to acknowledge them. They may not even be aware that they are doing this or, if they are, may be very reluctant to admit it. There are many people, mainly women, who spend their lives looking after an elderly parent or an invalid spouse and, often, such patients feel guilty if they allow worry, anxiety or fatigue to show. But emotions have to have an outlet; if a natural outlet is denied them, they will find one of their own and cause psycho-somatic disease. Insomnia may often be an early sign of such bottled-up emotions and hypnosis can offer a gentle way of allowing the patient to release her feelings and accept them for what they are.

In a case such as this, the patient would be encouraged, under hypnosis, to talk about how she felt and would be allowed to express emotions such as anger and resentment that it was impossible for her to show to the person in her care. Gradually, she could be persuaded that expression of her emotions was not wrong but, on the contrary, was a perfectly natural reaction to circumstances. She would also be reassured that there was no disloyalty involved in her 'letting go' like this because, as a result, her relationship with the person she cared for would improve, so that they would both benefit. Finally, she would be taught how to recognize her emotions and how to deal with them, instead of bottling them up and allowing them to cause illness.

Anxiety does not always express itself simply as in-somnia. Some patients have sleep difficulties because when they do go to sleep they have nightmares. These produce a two-fold effect: not only do they disturb the patient's sleep, but they also make him dread falling asleep in the first place. When a patient is hypnotized, these dreams can be explored. The examination of any episode or theme that seems to recur frequently may give a clue as to the underlying anxiety. In such a case, the patient may be asked to re-experience the nightmare while he is in hypnosis, but will be reassured that, since he is consciously going to bring these frightening scenes into his mind, he will also be able to control them. He is aided in this by suggestions from the therapist. For example, if he frequently dreams that he is being chased by savage dogs, the therapist can ask him to look again at the animals and see them change into something less fearsome – friendly tabby cats, perhaps. A suggestion may then be given that, because the dream has now changed into something fairly innocuous, it will not recur or, if it does, it will be in its new form.

In addition, the patient may be asked to express what the dream means to him. Since the meaning is usually hidden somewhere in the subconscious mind, one of the techniques used in regression therapy may be necessary. The patient might be told that the symbolic meaning of a certain component of the dream will automatically come into his head while the therapist counts to five. Or he might be told that if he looks hard at whatever it is that frightens him in his dream, he will see what it really symbolizes. So, for example, if the patient was worried by conditions at work and was constantly being harried by his employer, the savage German shepherd that, in his nightmares, was forever barking and snapping six inches from his ankles might suddenly be seen as his boss shouting or complaining.

When a patient is told that something will 'automatically come into his mind', it is essential that he makes his mind blank, in order to allow the subconscious to produce whatever is relevant. However, many patients find it difficult to do this, with the result that their answers are not spontaneous but the result of conscious thinking. One way of getting over this problem is to use the 'ideomotor' finger signalling technique. This means that it is the fingers that do the talking. The patient is asked to concentrate on the word 'yes' and is told that, as he does so, one of his fingers will start to lift up. When this has happened, the formula is repeated with 'no', 'I don't know' and 'I don't want to tell you'. Then the patient is told that a series of questions will be asked which he will not even have to listen to or concentrate on. His fingers will do the work for him and he can just lie back and relax. It is important, of course, that the therapist remembers which finger is which! One drawback to this technique is that all the ideas have to come from the therapist and, although it can be useful when he has a fairly clear picture of the cause of the problem, it can result in rather slow progress when the origins are obscure. Of course, finger signalling is not useful solely in cases of insomnia, but can be used in the treatment of a variety of patients with whom it is necessary to delve into the background of their complaints.

With some patients, it seems as though there is no deep-seated cause for their insomnia. For them, inability to sleep is just a habit. It may have started at a time when they were anxious or excited about something and the insomnia may have added to their anxiety. Now, with the original cause long gone, they continue to worry about their insomnia and a vicious circle is set up whereby the anxiety produces insomnia which produces anxiety. If this vicious circle can be broken, the patient will once again be able to sleep normally. In this sort of case, hypnotherapy can produce dramatic results. Firstly, it can relieve the patient of his anxiety by allowing him to relax. He can be given suggestions that it does not really matter whether or not he sleeps because, even if he doesn't, he will not feel exhausted. This is perfectly possible, since a lot of the exhaustion he feels is due to his anxiety and the resulting muscle tension. Even if he is still getting fewer hours than he needs, that which he has should now be more restful.

In addition to breaking the vicious circle, hypnotherapy can be used to teach patients how to get to sleep. I have mentioned that in the moments before one goes off to sleep, one is in a state very similar to a hypnotic trance. Thus hypnosis is closely linked to natural sleep although, as we know, it is not itself a form of sleep. When I first started to take an interest in hypnotherapy I was at a lecture where someone asked, 'Is there any risk that the patient may not come out of a trance?' The lecturer explained that if this happens it is always because the patient consciously wishes to stay in the trance. He then continued this reassurance by saying, 'If a patient is left in trance, ultimately he will drift into a normal sleep from which he will wake in due course. So you mustn't worry that if you suddenly drop down dead from a cardiac arrest something terrible will happen to your patient – he'll just go off to sleep and then wake up in due course – although not, unfortunately, in time to administer heart massage to his therapist!' So drifting from hypnosis into sleep is a perfectly natural phenomenon. Indeed, it is not unusual for a patient who is practising self-hypnosis to fall asleep on the odd occasion when he is feeling tired – and it is not unknown for an overtired patient to fall asleep during a session of hypnotherapy in the consulting room!

Thus, in the treatment of insomnia, the patient may be told that if he uses self-hypnosis at night when he is ready to go to sleep, he will automatically drift from a hypnotic trance into a natural sleep. He may find it difficult at first but, if he practises regularly, he will find that he can go to sleep very quickly whenever he wants to. And the great advantage of this method, compared with the use of sleeping tablets, is that if he should wake during the night he can use it again – and, of course, he will feel no 'after-effects' in the morning.

Anxiety

Anxiety lies at the root of many of the problems that are amenable to treatment with hypnosis. However, in many cases, it is the anxiety itself which is the main symptom. The patient will be aware of feeling anxious and tense all the time, even if she (or, less frequently, he) has nothing to be anxious about. Any upset in the daily routine, however minor, will add to the anxiety, and what might appear to the outsider to be a relatively trivial problem may seem to the patient to be insurmountable and may cause a considerable worsening of her symptoms. Usually, the patient knows that there is no real cause for her anxiety and as a result she worries about the way she feels, which, on the one hand, seems senseless, but on the other seems to be in complete control of her. This knowledge that the way one feels or acts is irrational is classic of the conditions described as neuroses in medical terminology. And, sometimes, the awareness of the irrationality of her behaviour can lead the patient to believe that she must be going mad. However, patients who are suffering from the more severe mental conditions known as psychoses (those who, in the old days, were labelled 'mad') have no insight into their conditions and can see nothing irrational in their own behaviour. The difference between the two groups has been succinctly, if rather light-heartedly, summed up by 'The psychotic believes that two and two make five; the neurotic knows that two and two make four – but worries about it.'

Psychotic patients cannot be helped by hypnosis and may be harmed by it. Since it may sometimes be difficult to diagnose cases which lie on the borderline of psychosis, it is important that any patient who wishes to have treatment from a hypnotherapist for a purely mental condition should consult either a doctor or a psychologist who specializes in the therapy and who will know whether or not hypnosis should be used. Some patients who have neuroses should also avoid hypnotherapy. These are people who are suffering from depression. They very often have, in addition to their depression, a degree of anxiety which, it might be thought, could benefit from treatment under hypnosis. However, if one thinks of the depression and the anxiety as two sides of the same coin, two aspects of the same illness which balance each other, it can be seen that if one removes the anxiety there is a good chance that the depression may get worse. One can think of the anxiety as being the element of the illness that stimulates the patient to keep going – remove it and he may lapse into deepest gloom. The harm that hypnosis may cause to such patients is one reason why doctors and other qualified hypnotherapists are always concerned about the use of hypnotism as an entertainment. It is vital that the hypnotherapist knows as much as possible about his patients before he starts to hypnotize them, so that those suffering from depression or psychoses may be directed elsewhere for treatment. But it is quite possible for such patients to find themselves acting as volunteers for hypnotic entertainments where the hypnotist knows nothing about them and may inadvertently make their condition worse.

However, for patients who are suffering solely from anxiety, without any coexistent depression, hypnotherapy can be extremely helpful. But, here again, it is advisable to consult a doctor or psychologist, since the symptoms of clinical depression (that is, the illness called depression) are different from the feeling of simply being depressed. So it may not be easy for the patient herself to judge whether she is suffering from anxiety alone or from anxiety plus depression.

In the past, patients who suffered from anxiety and the associated tendency to panic attacks were severely incapacitated when it came to leading a normal life. Panic attacks can occur at any time or in any place, sometimes when the patient is away from home, perhaps shopping or visiting friends. Because these attacks are so overwhelming, the patient may become terrified that an attack might occur when she is away from the safety of her home, and may therefore avoid going out whenever possible. (This is distinct from the condition of agoraphobia, in which the patient knows what it is that makes her anxious – that is, going out of the house – and the sensation is more one of constant overwhelming fear at all times when she is out. Panic attacks often seem to have no particular precipitating factor and may occur just as easily at home as when the patient is out.)

Psychotherapy can be helpful for such patients but the treatment takes time and involves frequent visits to a specialist. However, with the advent of tranquillizers, general practitioners suddenly found that they were able to treat patients suffering from anxiety and many found relief from librium, valium and similar preparations before there was any indication that such drugs could become addictive. Unfortunately, a patient who remains on tranquillizers long term may find that they become less and less helpful in suppressing the symptoms as time goes on, so that the doses need to be increased, thus making the side-effects, such as lethargy and inability to concentrate, more pronounced. And once on tranquillizers, a patient may be very unwilling to come off them again. Even if she is aware that she feels bad while taking them, she is scared that she will feel ten times worse after coming off.

Hypnotherapy, fortunately, presents none of these problems. It has no side-effects and its effects do not wear off with time. And, unlike tranquillizers, which merely suppress the symptoms, hypnotherapy improves the state of the patient's mind so that she is no longer anxious. As it is a self-help therapy, the patient can progress at the rate which suits her best, using regular self-hypnosis, and may need to return to see the therapist only occasionally. It may even be helpful for patients who are trying to come off tranquillizers, although those who have been on them for a long time may be hard to hypnotize. (Probably homoeopathy is the treatment of choice for these patients.)

Anxious patients often say that they find it impossible to relax, no matter how hard they try. Of course, the very fact that they are *trying* to do so rather than just allowing themselves to, is probably one reason why they cannot. However, when one uses hypnosis, the word 'relaxation' need not even be mentioned. The induction of the trance and its deepening may involve counting, deep breathing or a visualization and it is on these that the patient concentrates. Thus she may suddenly realize that she has relaxed without having been aware of doing so. Sometimes one can actually see the muscles and the tension lines of a patient's face relax as she sinks into a trance.

Once she is in hypnosis, the treatment of the anxious patient consists primarily in giving her confidence in her ability to relax and in teaching her how to do so. Therefore, she will often be taught self-hypnosis and will be told that, since it is possible for her to relax while in a trance, it is just as possible for her to relax at other times. Suggestions may be given to her that she will start to feel very much more relaxed in her everyday life and that she will find it much easier to cope with the sorts of situations that have worried her in the past.

Specific techniques may be taught to a patient who suffers from panic attacks in order to enable her to cope with them. These are really just elaborations on the 'calm and relaxed' technique mentioned in Chapter Four, where it is suggested that repetition of the phrase will bring about the desired effect. However, such a repetition by itself may not be enough to control an acute panic attack. So it may be helpful if, in addition, the patient can be given something physical to do to relieve her symptoms. In one method, as soon as she feels the panic rising within her she clenches her fists very firmly and takes a deep breath. Then she 'feels the panic running from the brain and from the rest of the body into the arms and down into the clenched fists'. Once all the panic has 'collected in the fists' she breathes out quickly and, at the same time, flings open her fists to 'throw the panic away'. Although the patient does not have to be in a hypnotic trance when she uses the technique it must, of course, be taught to her while she is hypnotized so that her subconscious mind will automatically do what is required when she goes through the ritual. As with most hypnotherapeutic techniques, she will probably have to practise it a number of times before it is really effective. Once it is working, however, the efficacy of the technique will be reinforced by her confidence in it and the resulting feeling of security often prevents further attacks from occurring.

In addition to these methods of treatment, the usual ego-strengthening techniques are also used and if there is a specific factor which is causing the patient's anxiety, this will be explored. More will be said about this under 'Phobias' (page 129).

Asthma

Asthma is a condition which is almost invariably associated with anxiety. In many patients, the precipitating cause may be an allergic one (such as allergy to pollen) but, because being unable to breathe is so frightening, the feeling that an attack is about to start may result in a large and sudden build-up of anxiety. And this, in turn, may make what would have been a minor asthmatic attack develop into a major one. In some patients, anxiety itself can bring on an attack. Once again we have a vicious circle, with anxiety causing asthma which causes anxiety and so on. Therefore, if one can control the anxiety, one can also control the asthma.

Since asthma commonly affects children, it is fortunate that they are very good subjects for hypnosis. Opinions vary as to the age at which one can begin to use hypnosis and, to a great extent, it depends on the individual child. It is important that he is old enough to concentrate on what the therapist is saying and to co-operate in the treatment. Children of six or seven usually present no problems, but hypnotherapists who specialize in treating children may be happy to treat patients who are younger than this.

When the patient is a child, the therapist, before inducing hypnosis, will usually start by explaining what it is that happens to the body during an asthmatic attack. The role of fear in the development of an attack is stressed and the therapist will tell the child that he can be helped to overcome this fear and to control his body. The child must agree to have the treatment of his own free will in order for it to be beneficial. Usually, he will be treated in the presence of one of his parents, although some thera- pists like to treat children with the same condition (for example asthma or eczema) in groups. Even when patients are hypnotized in groups, it is still possible to treat them individually, since they can be told, 'You will remain absorbed in a pleasant daydream until I put my hand on your shoulder and call your name.' Thus each patient will pay attention only to the suggestions that are meant speci- fically for him. In this way time can be saved by using one induction and deepening technique for several pati- ents, without detracting from the quality of the treat- ment.

Much of the basic treatment for asthma is the same as

that for anxiety. The patient, whether adult or child, is taught how to relax and how to put himself into hypnosis. The techniques for self-hypnosis may be made simpler for children – for example, they may just be told to repeat a particular word or phrase a certain number of times. However, when a child is taught to hypnotize himself, the therapist must take extra precautions in addition to those normally used. For example, a young patient will be told that he will only be able to put himself into hypnosis when one of his parents is in the house and knows what the child is doing, that he won't be able to hypnotize himself to entertain his friends and that, if an adult calls him while he is in hypnosis, he will immediately wake up.

As well as being taught basic relaxation techniques, the asthmatic patient, adult or child, can be given a formula with which he can break the vicious circle of anxiety and worsening asthma. This may be something akin to the 'clenched-fist' technique mentioned in the section on anxiety. Thus the patient would be asked to imagine all the tension and tightness that he feels in his chest transferring to his fists, from where he can throw it away. Or he may be given a phrase to repeat, with the suggestion that, as he does this, his breathing will become easier and his muscles will relax. If he normally uses an inhaler and finds this helpful, he may be given the suggestion: 'As you repeat the phrase, you will feel just as though you have used your inhaler, knowing that the tightness is relaxing and that you are beginning to breathe normally again.' Some therapists will, while the patient is in hypnosis, get him to feel an attack coming on, feel the tightness, feel it becoming more difficult to breathe, and then use whichever technique he has been taught to relieve the attack. At first a patient may be loath to induce an attack, for fear that he will not be able to control it. However, having done so, it can be pointed out to him that if the power of his mind is strong enough to produce an attack just by thinking about it, then it can also alleviate an attack. Once he can control a self-induced attack under hypnosis, he will find it increasingly easy to control 'real' attacks.

If a patient is put into hypnosis or hypnotizes himself during an attack that has recently started, it will usually abate. Such treatment is a very good way of demonstrating the power of relaxation in the control of asthma.

A remarkable method of treating asthma in children was discussed in a paper read at the 9th International Congress of Hypnosis, held in Glasgow in 1982. The paper, by Dr Antonio Madrid of the University of San Francisco, described asthma as being like 'a child crying for his mother' and suggested that one cause of asthma could be a failure of bonding at birth. Bonding occurs – or should occur – immediately after birth, when the baby is put into the mother's arms and a loving relationship begins. If, however, the baby has to be put straight into an incubator, or if the mother rejects him (perhaps due to post-natal depression or to an emotional state resulting from a traumatic birth), or if she is ill and herself needs specialist care, this vital relationship may never get off the ground. Dr Madrid and his colleagues investigated the cases of a number of asthmatic children and noted those in which bonding at birth seemed not to have occurred. And then the mothers of these children were offered treatment.

It may sound extraordinary that treatment of the mother should affect the child's complaint, but this therapy certainly seems to work. The mother is regressed, under hypnosis, to the time of the birth and is taken through her labour and delivery, but seeing it 'through rose-coloured spectacles'. In the trance she experiences an easy birth, the baby is put into her arms immediately it is born, and she feels a warm, loving relationship beginning to develop. Sometimes some of the mother's distress at the time of the birth was due to the fact that her husband was unable to be present. If this was the case, she is asked to visualize him sitting by her, holding her hand and giving her encouragement. Having had this therapy, the mother, although still knowing consciously that there were problems when her baby was born, will at the same time feel as though none of the trauma happened and as though bonding did occur. The subtle difference that this therapy can make in the relationship between mother and child may be all that is needed to reduce or to stop the child's asthmatic attacks.

Migraine

Migraine is often thought of as being just a severe form of headache but, in fact, there is more to it than just pain. At the start of an attack, a patient may see flashing lights and, sometimes, may temporarily lose his sight. He may also develop a tingling or numbness in his face and mouth. It is usually after this that the headache begins. The pain is often one-sided and may be particularly severe in the region of the eye. Once the headache has started, the patient may vomit. Women who suffer from migraine may find that attacks are more likely to occur in the week before a period is due.

It is important for the therapist to take exact details of the patient's attacks, since the symptoms can vary considerably from one person to the next. Some have several visual symptoms before the onset of the headache, others have none; some always vomit, others seldom do; some have migraines frequently, others only two or three times a year; some have attacks that last for 24 hours or more, in others they last for only a few hours.

Relaxation and more specific techniques may both play a

part in the treatment of migraine. It is possible to suggest to a patient that his attacks will become less frequent and less severe as he becomes more relaxed, since tension may often be a precipitating factor. However, it is usual, in addition, to teach the patient a method by which he may cut short a migraine should it occur. A simple technique is for the patient to go into hypnosis and rest his hand against the area of his head that is painful. He is told that he will gradually feel warmth flowing from his hand into his head, and this warmth will soothe and relax him. Slowly, the warmth will grow until it begins to replace the pain. Eventually, he will no longer be aware of any pain in his head – it will all have been replaced by a comforting feeling of warmth which will remain after he wakes from hypnosis and will then gradually fade. But the pain will not return. This method may work surprisingly quickly and may be used in self-hypnosis, or by the therapist if a patient comes to see him during an attack. Even migraines that have been going several hours and that have become quite severe may respond, although, of course, if the patient was using the technique himself, one would expect him to have done so before the attack got to that stage.

The 'clenched-fist' technique which can be so useful in ridding the asthmatic patient of the spasm in his lungs can also be adapted for the treatment of patients with migraine. However, this is best used at the start of an attack, so the patient may be taught both this and the 'warmth' technique to cover all circumstances. It is necessary to explain to the patient that a migraine occurs when, for reasons best known to themselves, the blood vessels in the brain start to contract and then over-dilate. The contractions result in inadequate amounts of blood reaching the areas supplied by these vessels and this causes the visual symptoms and the tingling sensations experienced by some patients. When the blood vessels dilate, these symptoms disappear because the areas are now getting enough blood, but over-dilation creates pressure against the surrounding structures and this causes the pain. When a patient uses the 'clenched-fist' technique, he first shuts his eyes and visualizes his brain. He sees that the blood vessels running through and around it are all tight and constricted. Once he can picture this clearly, he clenches his fists very firmly to mirror the constriction in the blood vessels. Then, very gradually, he relaxes his fists and, as he does so, he pictures the blood vessels in his brain relaxing and returning to normal. When he is being taught this technique, the therapist will tell the patient that as he pictures it happening, and mirrors it with his hands, the blood vessels will actually relax and return to normal and will not rebound into over-dilation. Thus not only will the symptoms associated with the constriction disappear but those associated with the over-dilation will not develop. The instructions for this technique are, of course, given to the hypnotized patient, but he does not have to put himself into hypnosis in order to carry it out; thus it can be used under any circumstances, although if it is possible for him to go into a trance he may find it even more effective.

Skin Complaints

It might be thought that although a condition in which the symptoms are entirely functional, such as migraine, might be readily treatable by relaxation and suggestion, one which appears to be purely physical, such as a skin condition, would not respond. However, this is far from being the case and eczema and psoriasis may both respond extremely well to hypnosis.

Very often a patient who suffers from psoriasis will notice that if she (or, less frequently, he) becomes agitated or tense, her skin gets worse. Therefore, although the actual cause of psoriasis is not known, it is obviously, in part, a psychosomatic condition. Treatment consists mainly in relaxation therapy, coupled with suggestions that the patches of psoriasis will become smaller and smaller until they disappear completely. The patient may be asked to picture her skin gradually becoming clearer, and this is a visualization that she can use during self-hypnosis.

Eczema frequently occurs in children. The itching that is associated with it may be so severe that the child scratches himself until he bleeds. And the constant itch may make him extremely fretful and irritable. Obviously, this state of mind is not going to help the skin to heal, so, here again, relaxation is the key. When children are treated with hypnosis, no matter what the reason, it is particularly important that they should feel secure. Therefore suggestions are often given to them while they are in a trance to reassure them that they are safe, that their parents love them and care about them and that, with the help of the hypnotherapy, they will get well again. Suggestions may be given that the itching will become less intense. This is known as a negative hallucination and may also be used in the treatment of chronic pain. A positive hallucination is one in which the patient is made to feel, or see, something that is not there; a negative hallucination is one in which he can no longer feel, or see, something that is there. A moderate to deep level of trance is necessary to induce either type of hallucination, but fortunately most children are good subjects.

With children (and, of course, with adults too) the therapist needs to explain what is going to happen in terms to which the patient can relate. For example, the irritation may have been going on for so long that it may be impossible for a child with eczema to remember what it feels like for his skin not to be itchy, let alone imagine the sensation. It is important, therefore, for the therapist to find out whether there is anything that relieves the condition, even partially. Perhaps the child has been using a steroid cream with some relief. In such a case, when he is being taught a technique, he might be told that it will relieve the itching just as much as the steroid cream – and perhaps a little bit more. Once the therapy has started to take effect, suggestions can be given that his skin will feel a little better every day. Finally, when the irritation is only minimal, a suggestion that it will stop completely will be accepted by the child's subconscious mind.

Most children are imaginative and can visualize without trouble. In the treatment of eczema, a child may be asked to imagine that he is swimming in a warm pool in a lovely garden and that, as he swims, the warm water is helping his skin to heal. He is told to look down through the clear water and see that the rash is slowly fading.

One practitioner who specializes in the treatment of children suggests to those with eczema that they imagine that their hands are growing bigger and warmer. Once they have done so, they are asked to stroke the affected areas with their large, warm hands and are told that the heat will make more blood flow through the skin. The blood will carry with it the nutrition that the skin needs to get better. Then the children are asked to imagine their hands getting small and cold. Again they stroke the affected areas and this time they are told that the coldness will seal in the healing properties of the blood so that the skin will continue to improve, even after they wake up from hypnosis. Once they have learned them, either of these visualization techniques can be used by children when they practise self-hypnosis.

One of the most extraordinary stories concerning the treatment of a skin condition by hypnosis was published in the *British Medical Journal* in 1952 by Dr A. A. Mason under the title, 'A case of congenital ichthyosiform erythrodermia of Brocq treated by hypnosis'. This rare condition is one that the patient is born with (congenital), and causes a thick, fish-like (ichthyosiform) layer of hard scaly skin to form all over the body. The patient in question had had plastic surgery to try to remedy the condition but, unfortunately, the grafted skin had soon become affected. Dr Mason was working in the hospital to which the patient had been admitted and, being at that time relatively inexperienced in dermatology (the treatment of skin problems), was unaware that this condition was both rare and apparently untreatable. (In fact, to the uninitiated, it may look somewhat like an extremely severe form of psoriasis.) Being interested in hypnosis, he therefore suggested to the patient that he might like to have some hypnotherapy. The patient agreed and Dr Mason began to treat him. He concentrated at first on one arm and, within a week, the skin was beginning to lose its scaliness. After several weeks of treatment, the condition had been reduced to limited patches and much of the patient's skin was normal. There is no explanation at all as to why hypnotherapy should have helped in a case like this and, owing to the rarity of the condition, it has been impossible to do a trial on other cases.

Enuresis (Bedwetting)

Bedwetting is a common problem and can cause great stress in a family. Because it is known that tension may make the condition worse, parents are always advised not to punish the child but to reassure him that they know that it is not his fault. However, for a parent having to cope with a bedwetting child, this is not always easy. A mother who has to wash sheets five, six or seven times a week is apt to become short-tempered. Eventually she may start to feel that the child really could control himself if he wanted to and that either he is continuing to wet because he is too lazy to get up to go to the toilet or because, for some reason, he wants to punish her. If there are other children in the family, they may get upset by the situation. They may resent the fact that their mother is always irritable; if they share a room with the child who wets, they may object to the fact that it often smells of urine; and if the wetting makes it impossible for the family to go on holiday this is bound to cause tensions.

In a case like this, it may be necessary to treat both the mother and the child. The mother can be taught to relax so that she can cope better with the problem, and the child, who is frustrated and miserable due to his inability to stop wetting, can be given a technique whereby he can help himself. There are, of course, orthodox methods of treatment. The 'alarm' method is popular and effective for a lot of children. The mechanism is attached to the bed and, if it becomes damp, it rings a bell or buzzer. This means that the child is wakened at the very moment that he starts to urinate. Eventually, he becomes so used to waking when he wants to pass water that he can do so automatically without the aid of the alarm. However, some children do not react to the alarms but manage to sleep through them. Another orthodox method of treatment involves the use of the drug imipramine (Tofranil), which for some reason not fully understood seems to prevent the child from wetting. But, here again, it does not work for all children, and there are of course many parents who would rather have to wash sheets than have their children taking drugs for any length of time.

Up to the age of about six, there is still a good chance that the child will grow out of his habit, so children under this age are not usually treated by any method. A child of six or seven may be treated with hypnotherapy if he is well motivated and, on the whole, children with enuresis are.

They dislike the problem as much as their parents do and are just as anxious that they should be able to stop.

The keynote to the treatment of a child with enuresis is reassurance. While in hypnosis, he must be reassured that his parents love him, even though they may sometimes get cross with him; he must be reassured that the bedwetting is not his fault and that there is no reason for him to feel guilty about it; and he must be reassured that he will be able to stop in due course. He is told that there are many things that his body can do for itself without him having to think about them – things such as breathing and digesting food – but, whereas the lungs automatically know how to breathe and the stomach how to digest, the bladder has to learn how to control passing water. In his case, it has obviously learned what to do most of the time, because when he is awake he doesn't wet himself and he can go a long time without having to pass water. Now the treatment that he is going to be given will teach the bladder how to behave at night. Once it has learned, it will never forget.

The child is told that the reason he wets at night is because his bladder lets go of the water it is holding long before it is full. He is asked to think of his bladder as being like a balloon, able to stretch and stretch so that it can hold lots of water. He is asked to put a hand on his abdomen and to picture his bladder stretching. As he does so, he is told that he will start to feel that he wants to pass water. When the sensation starts, he is to say to his bladder, 'You're not full,' and this will remind it that it can stretch even more, so the feeling will go away. He is told that if he practises this when he is doing his self-hypnosis, his bladder will remember what a lot of water it can hold. And, because he is constantly reminding it, it will remember, even when he is asleep, that there is no need to pass water until it is full. As a precaution, he is told that if the bladder does become very full during the night, he will wake up and go to the toilet, rather than wetting the bed. Finally, he is told that his bladder is very clever and will probably start to learn what to do quite quickly, so within a short time he should be having many more dry nights.

Many children will be able to stop bedwetting using a simple technique like this. But some have deep-rooted reasons for continuing to wet and, with these, some form of hypnoanalysis may be necessary. This is not possible with young children, but with older children may reveal problems that have been suppressed and that are manifesting as bedwetting. When the patient is in his teens, enuresis is harder to treat. If the condition has continued to this age, there is usually some underlying reason why and this may be hard to elicit. Adolescents may be poor hypnotic subjects and therefore investigation of their anxieties and emotions may be difficult. In addition, there may be some secondary gain from the enuresis (in other words, the patient may actually be getting some sort of benefit from continuing to wet the bed) and he may not wish to stop. Even if one can discover the root cause, it is essential that the patient understands and acknowledges it, so that he can learn to express his emotions in another way.

Pain

The use of an induced 'negative hallucination' was mentioned in the section on eczema. This is a technique which is also very useful for the treatment of chronic pain. However, the use of hypnosis for pain control is fraught with danger and should not be used except by doctors and dentists. It is certainly not something that patients with an ability to do self-hypnosis should try for themselves. The danger is, of course, obvious when one thinks about it. If one routinely uses hypnosis to remove pain, then one may easily mask a potentially life-threatening condition, such as an inflamed appendix or an ectopic pregnancy (where the foetus is growing in one of the tubes instead of in the womb). The therapist must therefore be completely sure that the pain that he is treating is not of diagnostic significance (in other words, he must be certain that it is not being caused by anything that needs investigation) and he must also ensure that the patient, once taught to use the technique, will be unable to use it for any other type of pain.

As a general rule, children are not taught to use self-hypnosis to alleviate pain. Even though a post-hypnotic suggestion is given that the patient will only be able to use the technique under very specific circumstances, it is wise to take extra precautions. For adults, this entails explaining to them, when they are not under hypnosis, the dangers of masking undiagnosed pains. But children may be unable to understand this, or may not remember it, so it is best not to teach them the technique. However, it is perfectly possible for a dentist, for example, to use hypnosis on a child during treatment and thus lessen the need for local anaesthetic, without actually having to teach the child to control pain himself.

Even with adults, further safeguards are necessary. For example, a patient who suffers from migraine or from tension headaches may get a severe headache due to another cause (such as high blood pressure or a severe infection) and may misinterpret this symptom as being the headache from which he usually suffers. Masking this headache may lead to diagnosis, and therefore treatment, being delayed. When he is taught the technique, therefore, he will be told that it will only mask the pain for a few hours. If the pain is still there when the effect wears off, this may be an indication that he should see his doctor. This form of suggestion may also be used for patients who are taught self-hypnosis by their dentists. The removal of pain may be an extremely useful technique when you suddenly develop toothache at eleven o'clock on a Sunday night, but if you continue to control the pain rather than going to the dentist, you may end up with a very severely infected mouth.

One simple method of pain relief has already been mentioned in the section on migraine – that of replacing the pain with a feeling of warmth. A useful method for dental treatment approaches pain control from the opposite direction, based on the idea that numbness can be caused by cold. The patient is asked to imagine that next to his chair there is a bucket containing some water and a lot of ice. When he can picture it clearly, he is asked to put his hand into the bucket. The therapist then continues to talk to the patient, telling him how cold his hand is getting, how he is losing the feeling in it, and so on. Finally, the patient is told to take his hand out of the bucket and to pinch it with his other hand. In this way, he proves to himself that his hand is really numb, since he cannot feel himself pinching it. Then he is told to lift his hand and place it against that part of his mouth in which the dental treatment is to take place. Gradually, he will be aware that the numbness is transferring from his hand to his mouth, his hand regaining sensation while his mouth becomes just as numb as his hand was before. Thus, when the treatment is carried out, he will not feel it, any more than he was able to feel himself pinching his hand.

Another method, requiring even more detailed visualization, is one in which the patient is asked to imagine an old-fashioned telephone switchboard that represents his brain. Wires are plugged in all over the place, linking the brain to different parts of the body. And next to each wire socket is an on/off switch and a little light. If the switch is at 'on' the light is on, and if the switch is turned off, the light is off. Each switch has a label under it saying which part of the body it is connected to, and the patient is asked to look for the socket and switch connected to the painful area which is to be treated. If, for example, the patient has an ingrowing right toenail, he looks for a label saying 'right big toe'. Once he has found it, he is asked to make sure that it is the correct socket by checking that the switch and the light are on. To make the visualization more vivid, he is asked to say what colour the light is and what colour the wire is which is plugged into the socket. He is then asked to turn the switch off and unplug the wire, and is told that in doing so he has cut off the nervous link between his brain and his right big toe. Therefore it is impossible for any pain signals to get through to his brain and he will feel no pain in the toe.

The anaesthesia that a patient feels as a result of this technique will be very localized and it is therefore a useful alternative to a local anaesthetic in suitable patients. Another method is to suggest to the patient that he is having a local anaesthetic injected into the painful area. One might wonder why this method should be any better than actually giving a local anaesthetic but, as anyone who has had one will know, the anaesthetizing injection can itself be quite painful. When one visualizes having such an injection under hypnosis, one does not imagine the pain associated with it, but only the resulting numbness.

In order to be able to produce any form of hallucination, a patient needs to be able to go into a medium-depth or deep trance, so those who are 'light' subjects may be unable to develop a sufficient degree of anaesthesia for minor operations or dental treatment to be performed. However, the technique can still be useful. A moderate degree of numbness can prevent the injection of a local anaesthetic from being unpleasant and may reduce the amount of anaesthetic that is needed. Even patients who cannot develop any useful degree of anaesthesia may benefit from being told that 'although you may still feel the pain, it will not

worry or upset you'. This can be a very important suggestion since the emotional content of a pain can add greatly to
its unpleasantness. It is well known that some pains are
much more unpleasant than others, even though they may
be of equal intensity. It is perfectly possible for patients to
endure quite severe pain if the emotional aspect has been
removed.

A further benefit of hypnosis in the control of pain is,
once again, its ability to relax the patient. Very often
chronic pain may become a vicious circle, with the pain
making the patient tense and the tension making the pain
worse. If the patient can be taught to relax when he feels
the pain coming on, rather than tensing up, the pain may
be reduced dramatically.

Terminally ill patients may be treated quite safely with
hypnosis and thus avoid the side-effects of heavy medication with analgesic drugs, the doses of which may be
reduced. Patients who have intermittent pain may, if they
are capable of inducing a hallucination, be taught the
technique of time distortion, so that it appears to them that
time passes very quickly when they have the pain and slows
down again to normal in between attacks.

Tinnitus

Tinnitus, or ringing in the ears, is a most unpleasant condition, usually occurring in older patients and often associated with deafness. The patient is aware of a constant
buzzing, hum or other sound, sometimes predominantly in
one ear, which may be so distressing that it dominates his
life. Orthodox medicine has little to offer in the treatment
of tinnitus but, fortunately, other therapies, such as acupuncture, homoeopathy and hypnotherapy, may be able to
relieve the patient of his symptoms.

Once again the hypnotherapeutic treatment involves the production of a negative hallucination, and so it is less likely to be of use for those patients who are only capable of going into a very light trance. However, since a constant noise in the ears and an inability to hear well may be very demoralizing, ego-strengthening techniques may benefit any patient with tinnitus and this, of course, may be done at any depth of trance.

In the same way that a patient can be taught to remove pain, so the patient with tinnitus can be taught to remove the ringing. Since there is no danger involved in masking the noise, no time limit need be put on the effect and the patient can be taught to use the technique himself, so as to maintain the hallucination if it should start to wear off.

A useful method is to ask the patient to visualize an old-fashioned radio, with large knobs and dials. When he can see it clearly, he is told that it is this that controls his tinnitus. If he looks closely, he can see that the 'volume' knob is turned up high and the needle on the dial next to it is showing almost maximum volume. He is then asked to move the knob slightly, so that the noise in his ears increases a fraction and the dial moves up even further. When he has done this, he is asked to turn the knob back to where it was and hear the noise decrease. It is often easier to start with the positive hallucination of an increase in the noise before starting to try to decrease it. Once the patient has got the tinnitus back to where it was originally, he is asked to start to turn the knob down very gently. It is important that this is done gradually to allow the patient to feel that he has complete control over what he is doing. At the first session, therefore, the tinnitus may be reduced slightly, but it may be some time before it is dispersed completely. However, if the patient is willing to practise his self-hypnosis regularly, he may find that it does not take long before the tinnitus is considerably reduced from its original level. Of course, as it decreases, the patient will gain confidence in his own ability to control the noise and this, in itself, will make the later stages of treatment easier.

It may be necessary for the patient to continue to do regular daily self-hypnosis for the rest of his life in order to keep a good control over his tinnitus, but most patients would consider this a small price to pay in order to get rid of this unpleasant complaint.

Phobias

A phobia is a condition in which the patient has an irrational fear of a particular thing and, although he knows that his fear is foolish, can do nothing about it. Mild phobias such as fear of spiders or mice are fairly common but it is usually possible to live with them. However, a severe phobia can disrupt the patient's life, since he spends all his time worrying about and trying to avoid the object of his fear. The commonest phobia for which treatment is requested is agoraphobia, or fear of open spaces, which may prevent the patient (usually a woman) from even being able to set foot outside her home. Then comes fear of illness or of death, followed by fear of other people or of animals. Other fairly common phobias are acrophobia (fear of heights), fear of the dark and claustrophobia (fear of small spaces). Less common ones include fear of water, of fire, of thunderstorms, of insanity, of snakes and of cats. And fear of doctors and dentists is not uncommon!

Hypnotherapy can be used in a variety of ways. Firstly, the patient must be given adequate ego-strengthening techniques, since the feeling that one's life is ruled by a ridiculous and unnecessary fear can be very demoralizing. He must be given confidence in himself and in his ability to conquer the phobia. Sometimes he may be taught to overcome his phobia by simple visualization techniques. For example, if the patient is a woman with agoraphobia who is unable to go outside her house without feeling panic, she might be asked to visualize herself inside her front door and about to open it. Very slowly, she opens the door and stands looking out but not stepping over the threshold. The hypnotherapist reassures her that she is quite safe, she is still in her house, she can shut the door at any time she wants to. He may give her a technique with which she can rid herself of any tension or anxiety which is beginning to build up. This may be something like the 'clenched-fist' technique mentioned in the section on anxiety, in which the patient can throw away her tension with her hands and breathe it out from her lungs. Or it may be a phrase which she can repeat to herself, such as 'calm and relaxed' or 'safe and secure'. Once she can picture herself standing at the open door without feeling any tension, she is asked to step out of the house. Again she stops and controls any tension or anxiety before going further. Next, she may take two or three steps, stopping only if she feels anxious. Going this slowly, it may take quite a long time before the patient can even get to her own garden gate, but all the time her confidence will be increasing.

Here again, self-hypnosis is very important and the patient must practise regularly. In order to give her added confidence when she is using the technique on her own, she may be told that if she feels anxious the visualization will stop just as if she has stopped a film from running. Not only will she stay still, but she will find that her anxiety is cut short. She can then use whatever technique she likes to ensure that she is relaxed and can start the film running again, either from where she was or else, if she prefers, from the beginning.

The more often the patient visualizes herself doing and coping with the action which previously brought on uncontrollable panic, the more confident she will become that she can do it in real life. She begins to have faith in her relaxation techniques and is told by the therapist that when she confronts her phobia they will work just as well as they do when she is in hypnosis. It is often a slow process, but patients who were previously unable to get out of the house may eventually be able to enjoy a normal life again.

In some cases, the patient may not respond, possibly because the phobia resulted from some very traumatic incident whose memory is still being stored, but suppressed, by the subconscious mind. In cases like this, it is necessary to undertake some form of hypnoanalysis to try to discover the original cause of the phobia. The techniques used are similar to those mentioned in the chapter on regression and, indeed, regression may be very helpful in the treatment of phobias.

The Use of Hypnosis in Obstetrics

There is no doubt that a woman who has attended ante-natal relaxation classes is far more likely to have an easy labour than one who has not. Ideally, the mother should be able to relax between contractions and, during the second stage of labour, should be able to use her contractions so that she pushes with them and does not struggle against them. It follows, therefore, that the relaxation induced by hypnosis should be of benefit to a mother in labour. However, hypnosis has far more to offer a pregnant woman than mere relaxation.

In recent years, paediatricians have become increasingly concerned about the effect on the newborn baby of pain-killing drugs given during labour. Mothers, too, have been aware of this problem and many have opted for 'natural childbirth'. However, even when a woman is fully prepared for her labour, she may still need to take pain-killers. But a patient using hypnosis may be able to control her pain so that she can either do without drugs altogether or make do with a very small dose. She will, of course, need to start her hypnotherapy sessions fairly early on in her pregnancy so that, by the time she goes into labour, she has had adequate practice in the various techniques that she will need to use. She will not be taught to anaesthetize her pain completely but will be told that any pain that she does feel during labour will not worry her. This last suggestion is very important. One of the complaints which may be expressed by women who have had an epidural for labour (an injection into the spinal column which anaesthetizes all of the body below the level of that injection) is that they did not feel that they were taking part in the delivery of their children. If pain is completely absent, then the work seems to have been done entirely by the midwives and the mother is left feeling vaguely unsatisfied and as though she has somehow missed out on this important experience.

It is, of course, important that someone should be present at the delivery who can help the mother with her hypnosis. Some hypnotherapists invite the midwife to attend the ante-natal hypnotherapy sessions so that she can give the appropriate instructions and suggestions when the patient is in labour. Some obstetricians practise hypnosis and offer it to their patients. The main problem with using hypnosis is that it is time-consuming for the hypnotherapist who has to run the ante-natal sessions. However, it would seem that this is time well spent when mothers come through their deliveries with ease and when the risk of their babies being affected by sedatives and pain-killers is removed.

The Use of Hypnosis in Dentistry

Hypnosis has several uses in dental practice. It can be used to calm patients who are afraid to have treatment; it can be used to produce analgesia; and suggestions can be given that the time the patient has to spend in the dentist's chair will seem to pass very quickly.

When treating people who have a phobia about going to the dentist, it is probably advisable to see them, for the first few sessions at least, outside the dentist's surgery. Many dentists now use hypnosis and may have a separate room in which they can treat patients of this kind. Otherwise, the patient may be treated by another hypnotherapist and passed on to the dentist once the fear of entering the surgery has been reduced. The treatment of this problem is along the same lines as that of other phobias. The dentist himself does not need to be a hypnotherapist. Like Dr Bramwell (mentioned in Chapter Two), the therapist has only to tell the dentist the key phrases necessary for him to be able to put a 'primed' patient into hypnosis and, once in a trance, the patient can do the rest.

.For a patient who wishes to avoid having injections for dental treatment, the numbing effect of the 'hand in the bucket of ice', described in the section on pain, can be used. The numbness of the hand is then transferred to the appropriate section of the jaw. Since this technique may take quite a time before complete analgesia occurs, the dentist, or other hypnotherapist, would probably teach the patient how to use self-hypnosis and allow him to practise at home for a few weeks before coming for treatment.

CHAPTER SEVEN

SOME CASE

HISTORIES

Much of life is a learning process and the way that one's mind reacts today depends very much on what experiences one has been through in the past. A child who has burnt his fingers on a match will have learned that naked flames are painful. Similarly, a child who has been shut into a small cupboard may have 'learned' that enclosed spaces are frightening. In order to treat abnormal mental or psychosomatic states in the present, it may be necessary to dig up the past. In this respect, hypnotherapy can be very challenging because the therapist must know not only how to bring important information to the fore but also how to deal with it. And, of course, one never knows what is going to come up. No two patients ever respond in exactly the same way to hypnosis because no two patients are identical. Even if they have had very similar traumatic experiences or, indeed, have lived through the same traumatic experience, the effect on them will not have been the same. When hypnoanalytic treatment is necessary, the patient will probably need quite a long period of therapy before he is completely better. But whichever techniques are needed, it is impossible to tell a patient in advance how long his treatment is likely to take. However, if, after three to five sessions, there is no sign at all of any progress, he should probably think about trying a different therapy.

The cases related in this chapter are all actual case histories and show how varied can be the results of hypnotherapy.

Mr R. S.

Mr R. S. was a policeman who had failed his promotion examinations on two occasions. Now he was very anxious in case he failed a third time, since that would probably mean that he would not be allowed to re-take them. One particular subject in the examination worried him and he found that his anxiety made it impossible for him to retain much information about it.

The initial treatment was to teach him to use hypnosis as a form of relaxation. He was taught how to put himself into hypnosis and was told to do this every day for 15 minutes before he started his revision. He was told that if he repeated the formula 'calm and relaxed' several times every 15 minutes or so while he was studying, he could stop himself from becoming tense. If tension did begin to build up, he could get rid of it by taking a deep breath and breathing the tension out. He was given several ego-strengthening suggestions and was told that there was no reason why he should not pass these exams – it was only his anxiety that was holding him back, not his capability.

Once he had practised these techniques and was beginning to take a more relaxed attitude towards his studies, Mr R. S. was told that if he recorded onto tape the things that he wanted to learn and played it to himself while he was under hypnosis, he would retain a great deal of the information. He started to use this method and was able to pass his exams without difficulty.

Mrs L. J.

Mrs L. J. was 42 years old and had been suffering from psoriasis for about seven years. The condition was not very bad but she always wore long sleeves and thick stockings to cover the unsightly patches which were noticeable on her elbows and legs. She also had some involvement of her scalp, so that she appeared to have an unpleasantly heavy dandruff. Originally only her elbows and knees had been affected, but in the past two years larger areas had become involved. Her mother had quite a severe form of psoriasis and Mrs L. J. was worried that hers, too, would become widespread.

Although not a naturally anxious person, there were some stresses in Mrs L. J.'s life. She admitted that there was sometimes tension between her husband and herself. He was an executive in a large company and often came home late, tired and bad-tempered. She had a fairly demanding part-time job and had two young children so that she, too, was often tired by the time her husband arrived home. She sometimes had to 'bite her tongue' in order to avoid arguing with him, but would then seethe inwardly because she hadn't told him what was on her mind. She was very much aware that the resulting tension or any other emotional stress would make her psoriasis worse. When she went on holiday, however, her skin got much better.

She was treated with the usual techniques of ego-strengthening and was taught to hypnotize herself. She was told that she would become very relaxed in everyday life, able to cope easily with everything that she had to do and that minor traumas would not upset her. She was told that gradually even her skin would relax and this would allow it to obtain more nourishment from the blood and to heal itself. She was asked to do regular self-hypnosis, in which she was to visualize the patches of psoriasis becoming smaller and smaller until they eventually disappeared.

At her second appointment, Mrs L. J. reported that she had been practising self-hypnosis every day and was feeling more relaxed. However, she didn't feel that she was going very deeply into hypnosis when at home. Despite this, she continued to improve, becoming far less tense. She began to realize that some of the tension at home had come from her, and now that she was more relaxed, her husband seemed less bad-tempered. She had five sessions of hypnotherapy, at intervals of about ten days, after which her psoriasis had completely disappeared. She was asked to continue with her self-hypnosis every day, visualizing her skin remaining clear and unblemished, and to return if she had any problems. She returned once, eight months later, when a very small patch of psoriasis had appeared after an emotional upset. This disappeared after one session and the therapist did not see her again.

Mr P. S.

At the outbreak of the Second World War, Mr P. S. was 21 years old and was called up into the Army. He was an intelligent and capable young man and soon rose to the rank of corporal. However, his Army service was cut short when he was badly injured in action. He was in hospital for several months and eventually had to have his right leg amputated.

Being young and resilient, he soon learned to walk with a prosthesis (false leg) and even managed to go dancing again, although he missed being able to play football. Soon after the war ended, he found a job with a firm in the City of London and slowly worked his way up the ladder until, in 1972, he became a director of the company.

After his leg was amputated, Mr P. S. had intermittent pain in the stump. For many years this was not very bad, but in the ten years before he had hypnotherapy it had started to get much worse. It would come on if he had walked a great deal and would sometimes appear when he was relaxing in the evening after a busy day.

He lived in Sussex, near the coast, and therefore had to

commute to London on the train every day. Sometimes he was not able to get a seat on the train to London Bridge, nor on the underground which took him to the City. He then had a six-minute walk to his office which meant that he often arrived in great pain. And the same thing might happen on the way home in the evening, although he was inclined to leave work late in order to miss the worst of the rush-hour.

Over the years, Mr P. S. had consulted his GP frequently about the problem. He had been back to the Limb Centre at Roehampton on numerous occasions and various types of prosthesis had been tried, but none seemed better than any other. He had been referred by his GP to see a surgeon and a neurologist but no one had been able to help him. He was given pain-killers to take if he needed them but he tried to avoid doing so when he was at work, since he was afraid that they might impair his concentration (although he had to admit that there were times when the severity of the pain made his mind wander).

He described the pain as being cramp-like and he was aware that he would get it more often when he was par- ticularly busy or under pressure at work. It could come on quite suddenly and, on occasion, would last for two or three days. In the past six months he had been having it every day and it was gradually getting more and more severe. When he took pain-killers, he no longer found them as helpful as they had been in the past. The pain was not associated with any soreness or redness on the skin surface and was obviously due to some form of muscle spasm and not to an ill-fitting prosthesis. (The pain from which Mr P. S. was suffering was not the same as the phenomenon of 'phantom limb pain' which is well known in amputees. The latter usually occurs immediately after the amputation and seems to the patient to be coming from the limb that is no longer there, often from the farthest part, the foot or the

hand. This type of pain, too, may be treated with hypnotherapy and, in a trial conducted in the 1950s, over 80
per cent of patients had relief from pain, although the effect
was long-lasting in only about 50 per cent.)

Finally, at his GP's suggestion, Mr P. S. decided to try
some hypnosis, although he was doubtful as to whether it
could help. However, on the grounds that it couldn't do
any harm, he made an appointment. Fortunately, he was a
good hypnotic subject and was capable of getting easily
into the depth of trance necessary to induce pain relief. At
his first session the therapist taught him how to hypnotize
himself and asked him to practise this every day for two
weeks before returning for his second appointment. He
was also taught a variation of the 'clenched-fist' technique
used for asthma, in order to relieve some of the spasm that
was occurring in the muscles of the stump.

At the second session, Mr P. S. reported that he had
been determined to allow the therapy to work if it possibly
could and had practised his self-hypnosis quite successfully
for about three days. But then, for some reason, he had
'lost the knack' and, although continuing to practise, had
been unable to put himself into a trance. It seemed as
though the reason for this was that he did not yet have
adequate confidence in his ability to use the techniques
that he had been taught, and so these were repeated. In
addition, the 'telephone switchboard' visualization technique (mentioned in the section on pain relief) was tried.
Mr P. S. found it hard to visualize the switchboard but
agreed to practise for a week to see whether it became
easier (as often happens). Unfortunately, although it did
become somewhat easier over the week for him to visualize
the switchboard and to 'turn off' the appropriate link to his
leg, this only eased the pain slightly. Therefore, at his next
session, the 'bucket of ice' technique (also mentioned in the
section on pain relief) was tried and he found this much

easier. As soon as his hand went numb, he was asked to place it on his stump, over the painful area. He was given suggestions that the numbness would leave his hand and flow into the stump, deadening the pain, while his hand would return to normal. The smile that developed on his face showed the therapist that the suggestion was taking effect.

Because there was no danger involved in masking this pain permanently, Mr P. S. was told that the effect would be long-lasting but that, if he felt that it was wearing off, he could 'top it up' by repeating the technique. It was suggested that he might routinely go through the technique two or three times a week, while doing his self-hypnosis, in order to maintain the analgesic effect at a constant level. However, although there was no danger in deadening this pain, there was always a possibility that other pains might occur in his stump, perhaps because of the skin being rubbed by the prosthesis, or caused by an infection. Therefore the therapist added, 'This is a very special kind of numbness. It will deaden only the pain from which you have been suffering for so many years, and on that it will be very effective. However, it will have no effect whatsoever on any other pain that occurs in the stump. Nor will it have any effect on any pain occurring anywhere else in your body.' When Mr P. S. woke up from the hypnotic trance he said that the pain had gone. He was asked to return in two weeks.

After this session he was able to control the pain quite successfully. He found that it was reduced by the initial relaxation and what remained was then fairly easily removed by the 'ice bucket' technique. However, once again he seemed to lose confidence in himself after about five days and was no longer able to control the pain, although he could still put himself into hypnosis. When he came for his next appointment, the techniques that he had learned previously were reinforced and he was given additional suggestions that he would begin to feel very confident in his ability to use them.

Three weeks later, he returned in a very jubilant state. He had had hardly any pain since his last session of hypnosis and that which had occurred he had been able to 'knock on the head' by using the 'ice bucket' technique. His only complaint was that he hadn't discovered hypnotherapy sooner!

Mr P. S. had only one more session of treatment. This was about two years later, when he requested an appointment to reinforce what he had previously been taught. He had been very busy during the past few months and had allowed his self-hypnosis to lapse. The pain had just started to come back and he was a little concerned in case he had lost the knack of dealing with it. However, when he went for his appointment, it was clear to the therapist that he was still perfectly capable of controlling the pain, but just needed to be reassured that this was the case and to be encouraged to practise his self-hypnosis as often as he could.

Mrs J. S.-C.

Mrs J. S.-C., who was 26 years old, went to a hypnotherapist 'as a last resort' to try to get some relief from a painful back. She had had the problem for about six years, following an episode when she had strained herself while doing some heavy lifting. The pain had recurred at frequent intervals and, in the last three years, the episodes had become longer and the pain-free periods between had become shorter. When she was in pain, she found that she was unable to do housework, cooking or shopping. Sometimes she was incapacitated for a week or more and she became very distressed when she had to rely on her husband to do the things which she felt were her responsibility. They had been married for three years and would have liked to have started a family but Mrs J. S.-C. felt that she could not face going through a pregnancy in her present state of health. In addition, she had started to believe that eventually she would have the pain constantly and would be confined to a wheel-chair, in which case she would be quite unable to look after a family. She longed to be more active but, even in between attacks, she was extremely careful about what she allowed herself to do, for fear that the pain would start up again.

Soon after she first strained her back, Mrs J. S.-C. saw her GP and was referred for some physiotherapy. She found this helpful to begin with, but after the pain had recurred for the third or fourth time, physiotherapy no longer seemed to have any effect. Some three or four years later she tried osteopathy, but did not find it helpful.

When she first went for hypnotherapy, she was taking a considerable number of pain-killers on a regular basis. She said that as soon as the pain started she could feel herself becoming tense because she 'knew' that she was going to have several days of severe pain. She was inclined to be a worrier and, for a year or two, had been suffering from tension headaches which had been getting more frequent and now occurred about once a week. As the therapist listened to her talk, it became clear to him that what was uppermost in her mind was the fear that she would be confined to a wheel-chair and in constant pain for the rest of her life. He began to wonder whether it might be possible to do more for her than just give her a technique to relieve the pain, since, if tension was contributing in a large part to the pain, teaching her to relax should help to relieve it. However, since she had had so little relief from other therapies, there was some doubt as to whether hypnosis could make her entirely better again.

Fortunately, Mrs J. S.-C. was a good subject and went into hypnosis readily. After the initial deepening and ego-strengthening techniques, she was given suggestions that she had nothing to fear – her back would not get worse and she would not finish up in a wheel-chair. She was told that she was in the process of learning to relax and that being able to do this always made life easier. Even if she was not free of pain, the very fact that she could relax would make it easier for her to cope and to carry on with her life. She was taught self-hypnosis and then a progressive relaxation technique. This technique is sometimes used to deepen the patient's trance at the start of a session and is one which people commonly use, without hypnosis, to help them get to sleep. There are several versions, but in this case Mrs J. S.-C.'s therapist asked her to imagine that a flood of golden light was pouring down onto the top of her head and was flowing down through her body and around it, bathing her with warmth and relaxation. As she did so, he asked her to concentrate on each group of muscles in turn and feel them relax, starting with the muscles of the scalp, then the forehead, the face and the jaw. (Good subjects may drop the jaw to such an extent that the movement can be seen by the therapist sitting several feet away.) Then he asked her to concentrate on the muscles of her neck, feeling them relax as they were bathed in the golden light. After this, he turned her attention to her shoulders (usually tense, even in the most relaxed person) and her arms and asked her to imagine that she was becoming loose and floppy like a rag doll. She was told to relax all the large muscles of the chest and, here again, the effect may be visible to the therapist. In normal breathing, the chest cavity is made larger and smaller by the movement of the muscles of the chest wall and by the diaphragm, a large sheet of muscle which divides the chest from the abdomen. When we are completely relaxed, we breathe just with the diaphragm and one can sometimes see this change to diaphragmatic breathing when the patient consciously relaxes the chest muscles.

Because she was already anxious about her back, there was the possibility that mention of it and a suggestion to relax it might make Mrs J. S.-C. more tense rather than less. Therefore the therapist just asked her to feel the warm golden light flooding over her back, soothing it and making it more comfortable, without suggesting any attempt at relaxation on her part. She was asked to feel herself sinking into the chair, the use of the word 'sinking' also implying that the patient will go deeper into the trance. Finally, she was asked to relax the muscles of her abdomen and of her legs and feet.

Once she had gone through this progressive relaxation, the therapist suggested that Mrs J. S.-C. should just sit and enjoy being in hypnosis and then asked her whether she felt any different from before. After a few moments she said that the pain, which had been quite bad when she arrived for her appointment, was slightly less. This gave something on which he could base his next suggestions. He told her that the reason that the pain had eased slightly was because she was more relaxed than she had been previously. He reminded her that, earlier, he had said that learning to relax would help to relieve the pain and, already, she was seeing that this was true. (In fact, he had not told her this – what he had said was that learning to relax would help her to cope with the pain, which is rather different. However, as it now seemed that relaxation was going to relieve the pain, the suggestion could be changed. Fortunately, it is possible to do this in hypnosis without troubling the patient, who will usually accept the most recent statement as being accurate.)

The therapist went on to tell Mrs J. S.-C. that a part of her pain was due to spasm in the muscles of the back. It might be a large part or a small part – only time would tell. But, since spasm could be relieved by relaxation, and since, with practice, she would learn to relax enough to get rid of all the spasm, there was no doubt that she would be able to relieve part of her pain. The spasm, she was told, was part of a vicious circle. When the pain started she became tense and anxious, because she was worried that she would not be able to look after her home and her family, and she was scared that this time the pain would be here to stay and she would finish up in a wheel-chair. The tension and the anxiety naturally made themselves felt in the place where she was most susceptible – in her back. And so, the more worried she got, the more spasm there was in her back muscles – and this worried her even more. Now that she knew that some of the pain was due to spasm, and that by relaxing she could relieve the spasm and reduce the pain, there was no longer any need for her to get tense or anxious when the pain came on. She was told that the relaxation would also help to control her headaches, which, as she knew, were due to tension.

Finally, the therapist taught her a variant on the 'clenched-fist' technique used for treating migraine. He suggested that as soon as the pain came on – either in her back or her head – she lie down, shut her eyes, clench her fists tightly and then very slowly relax them, visualizing, at the same time, the relaxation of the back or head muscles that had gone into spasm. She should then follow this up by visualizing the golden light and using the progressive relaxation technique. The therapist recommended that she practise her self-hypnosis at least once a day, or more frequently if she had time, and that, on each occasion she go through the progressive relaxation technique. He made an appointment to see her again in two weeks.

When Mrs J. S.-C. returned, the therapist asked first about her headaches, since it seemed likely that the minor ailment might have responded to treatment even if there had not yet been an improvement in her back pain. She said that she had had two, one of which she had been able to control. He told her that this seemed to be an encouraging start and then asked whether she had noticed any improvement at all in her back. 'Oh, yes,' she said. 'It's much better.' She had had one attack of sciatic pain since her last session. When it started, she didn't have her usual feelings of anxiety and distress and was able to control it with the techniques that she had been taught. She said she had been waking up each morning with some pain in her back, but this wore off once she was up and about.

The therapist hypnotized her again and repeated the suggestions that he had given to her on the first occasion. He told her that, since she had mastered these techniques so quickly, she would find that she could control her pain, even if it came on at a time when she could not lie down and practise her progressive relaxation. In future, just by visualizing the golden light flowing over her back, she would be able to relax the muscles and reduce the pain. She was told that from now on her back muscles would be as easy to control as her hand muscles or her face muscles. She could control her hands perfectly for writing, sewing, and so on, and her face for speaking and eating. The back muscles were no different and therefore there was no reason why she should not be able to control them just as well.

Mrs J. S.-C.'s third appointment was a month later. She reported, with delight, that she had had nothing more than some mild backache after doing heavy housework. She was now quite convinced that she would not finish up in a wheel-chair and this, in itself, had relieved a considerable amount of tension. She also noticed that she was feeling very much more relaxed in herself and that she was coping very much better with situations which, previously, would have made her nervous and panicky. The therapist suggested that if she had any more twinges she might return to see the osteopath since, now that the spasm was dealt with, he should be able to restore her back to a state in which she would be totally free from pain.

A year later, Mrs J. S.-C.'s husband phoned to say that she remained well and had just given birth to a baby girl.

Mrs R. G.

Mrs R. G. was 31 years old and happily married with three children aged ten, seven and four. She initially went to see a hypnotherapist because she wanted some help in her attempt to lose a stone in weight. She was given suggestions that she would not become hungry between meals and that she would be able to resist eating sweet foods and fatty foods. She was asked to project herself forward to the time when she would have lost the weight and to see herself looking in a mirror, admiring her new figure. Because she was very keen to slim, the suggestions were rapidly effective and she found she was able to keep to the diet that she had set herself without any desire to break it. Within a month she had lost her target amount and was very pleased with herself. Having reported her success, she went on to ask the therapist whether he could treat her seven-year-old son, who suffered badly from asthma. The therapist explained that with seven-year-olds a lot depended on their ability to concentrate, and that, although one could never guarantee results, it was possible that hypnotherapy might help.

He asked Mrs R. G. about her reactions to the asthma attacks – sometimes a parent can become so anxious that this in itself can make the child worse. However, she was a sensible woman and she said that she took the attacks in her stride, administering the medication prescribed by the doctor and calling him in if the attack seemed to be getting bad. 'It's upsetting to see Peter like that but I try to reassure him,' she said. 'Anyway, I have great faith in our GP, so that stops me from panicking.'

Asked about Peter's general health, Mrs R. G. said that he was a fairly sturdy little boy 'which is amazing really in view of the asthma and the fact that he had a difficult start to life'. On questioning, it turned out that Peter had been born prematurely and had spent the first four weeks of his life in an incubator. Mrs R. G. had not even been able to hold him until he was a few days old. From the first, Peter was fed with her milk, but she had needed to express it as he was too small to suck. And once she started to breast-feed him, it was a while before he was able to take enough from her. Although Peter was never in danger, his parents were both very worried about him and Mrs R. G. thought that they had never quite lost this anxiety. Despite the fact that she tried to be sensible about his asthma, she and her husband were both inclined to fuss more over Peter than over either of their other two children.

It sounded from the history as though bonding had not occurred at birth. Outwardly, this did not seem to have affected the relationship between Peter and his mother. However, from what she had said, it seemed very likely that Mrs R. G. and her husband, quite unconsciously, treated Peter in a different way from his brother and sister.

Regression to the time of Peter's birth, with a 're-telling' of the story, could subtly adjust Mrs R. G.'s attitude to him, both with regard to bonding and to her anxiety. When the technique was explained, she was keen to try it. Her GP had no objection to the treatment and so she made another appointment to see the therapist.

At the next session, Mrs R. G. was put into a hypnotic trance and techniques were used to get her as deep as possible. The object of the first part of the therapy was to make her subconscious mind accept the suggestion that Peter was not born at 34 weeks but at 38 weeks – in other words, only two weeks early. The therapist asked her to remember back to the day of her last appointment at the ante-natal clinic before Peter was born.

'Picture yourself going in and giving your name to the receptionist at the desk. I expect you know her quite well by now, don't you?'

'Yes – Mrs Jones. I see her sometimes in Sainsbury's.'

'She's crossing you off on her list, and she says that this may be your last appointment before the baby's born. A lot of the ladies deliver a week or two early, so, as you're now at 38 weeks, it could be any time now. Now go slightly further forward in time, until you're in the cubicle, waiting to see the consultant. Are you lying on the couch?'

'Yes.'

'What colour gown are you wearing?'

'Blue.' (Asking questions about details such as colours can help the visualization to become clearer.)

'And now the consultant's coming in. What's his name?'

'Mr Davidson.'

'He's asking how you are. What are you telling him?'

'I feel fine.'

'Good. And now he's going to have a feel of your tummy. He says the baby is a good size and is the right way up. It feels to him as though it could be due any time. He's very pleased with you. Everything's going very well. He tells you to get dressed and says that he will see you again next week if you haven't yet had the baby. Otherwise, he'll see you on the ward.'

Mrs R. G. was then asked to visualize further scenes in which hospital staff and friends commented on the fact that the baby must be almost due and that she would be going into hospital very soon. Having established that Peter's birth, when it occurred, was not going to be premature,

because she was 38 weeks pregnant, she was taken forward
to the time when her labour pains began. She was asked
how she felt when she realized that she was going into
labour and she said, 'Excited.' This was a good indication
that she had accepted the suggestion that Peter would not
be premature – if she had been anxious at going into
premature labour, she would have said 'nervous' or
'worried' rather than 'excited'. She was asked to re-live the
journey to the hospital, describing it as she went, and then
her admission into the labour ward.

Once again Mrs R. G. was taken forward in time, to a
point just a few minutes before Peter's birth. She was asked
to describe the midwives who were attending her and was
given suggestions such as, 'They're so kind, aren't they.
They make you feel so confident and happy.' She was told
that her husband was there by her side, holding her hand
(because it had been a premature birth in real life, her
husband had not been allowed to stay with her in case any
emergency procedures were necessary). Finally, she described Peter being born and starting to cry.

'And now the midwife has picked him up and wrapped
him in a towel and is handing him to you. Take him and
hold him. He's a lovely boy, fit and healthy. And you're so
happy. Your husband's there too and he's just as happy as
you are.'

In this way, Mrs R. G. was given an alternative story
which her subconscious mind could use to replace the
unhappy memories of the actual birth. She was told that, in
future, she would behave as though Peter's birth had been
just the way she had pictured it and she would no longer be
affected by any problems that might have occurred. When
she was woken up from the trance, Mrs R. G. was smiling
and happy.

Some weeks later she phoned the therapist to say that
although it was November, Peter's asthma had been much

less troublesome than usual. They had just been to see the specialist at the local hospital and he had been so pleased with Peter that he had reduced some of his medication. The therapist heard nothing more but, two years later, a chance meeting with Mrs R. G. in the street brought the story up to date. Peter, she said, was very well, doing well at school and taking part in sports. His asthma attacks occurred very rarely now and he no longer had to take medication all the time. The improvement, she said, dated from the 'bonding' session of hypnotherapy. Of course, some children do grow out of asthma and so one cannot claim all the credit for hypnotherapy. However, Mrs R. G.'s next remark was very interesting: she said, 'And since I had that hypnotherapy, Peter and I have become so much closer – I've got a really wonderful relationship now with all my children.'

Julia

The first hypnotherapy that Julia ever had was as an emergency. She was a talented 17-year-old dancer who was a full-time student at a ballet school and was hoping to dance professionally. Her school was putting on an evening of ballet excerpts and she had some important solos. However, at lunchtime on the day of the show, she started to develop a migraine. She had been suffering from migraines since the age of 14 and, recently, they had been getting more frequent. This was the second attack that she had had within four weeks. She had noticed that they were more likely to happen when she was nervous or under stress and she put the increased frequency down to the fact that she was studying for her A-levels as well as working hard towards a dancing career.

She was sent home from school to rest but by five o'clock

was no better. Her mother thought she would have to ring the school to tell them to put on an understudy but decided, first of all, to ring her GP to ask if there was anything he could give her that might help. The doctor's receptionist, on hearing what the problem was, put Julia's mother through to the young doctor who had recently joined the practice and who had trained as a hypnotherapist. He agreed to come out and see what he could do.

And so, at six o'clock, an hour and a half before the curtain was due to go up, Julia had her first session of hypnosis. She was complaining of a severe throbbing headache in the right side of her head. The light hurt her eyes and she was lying in a darkened room. Any movement or touch made her headache worse, so she lay very still, with her eyes shut. She had vomited twice. The doctor explained to her that if she followed the instructions that he gave her, there was a good chance that her headache would be relieved. An incentive such as this often helps to get patients into hypnosis if they are in pain. She went into a trance easily and was asked to lay her hand against the part of her head where the pain was most severe. She did so, gingerly. Then she was asked to feel the warmth from her hand flowing into her head and soothing away and replacing the pain. After about five minutes, during which time the suggestion was repeated several times, she started to smile and said, 'It's going.' After another few minutes she said, 'It's gone.' The doctor then woke her up, having told her that her headache would not return that evening.

Once awake, she was free of pain, although feeling a little weak. However, once she had had something to eat and drink, she felt well enough to go back to school and take part in the show.

Since Julia wanted to be a professional dancer, it was important that she should not be plagued by migraine every time she had an important role. She decided, therefore, to have some more hypnotherapy to try to get rid of the migraine for good. Having experienced rapid pain relief in the first session, she was very receptive to the idea that hypnosis was going to work and she went easily into a moderately deep trance. She was taught self-hypnosis and the technique, described in Chapter Six, in which a visualization of the blood vessels of the brain gradually relaxing their spasm is mirrored by a gradual relaxation of the clenched fists. She practised self-hypnosis regularly. Two weeks later, she returned for her next appointment and reported that a few days earlier she had been sitting watching television when she saw spots in front of her eyes and her vision became distorted – sure signs, for her, that a migraine was coming on. She immediately used the 'clenched-fist' technique. Within a few minutes she was free of symptoms and no headache developed.

Julia was seen once more, a month later, when she said she had had no further symptoms despite the fact that she was working very hard at present. Since she was still practising self-hypnosis every day, she was confident that if a migraine did start she could control it without problems.

Paul

This 14-year-old boy was taken to the surgery one morning by his mother. He had developed a large and painful abscess on his shoulder over the past few days and his mother had decided that medical treatment was now necessary. The boy looked glum and said that he had 'not wanted to bother the doctor', and that he was sure it would get better by itself. On examination, however, the abscess was a large one and in obvious need of being opened and drained. When Paul was told this, he went very pale and it became clear that his reason for 'not wanting to bother the doctor' was nothing to do with the conviction that the abscess would heal itself, but was solely due to the fact that he would rather have the abscess than the treatment.

The doctor told Paul that once the abscess had been incised he would feel a great deal better and that the procedure would be performed under a local anaesthetic. However, this was of little comfort to him since he was as scared of needles as he was of the incision, and anyway, he wasn't at all sure that the anaesthetic would work. By this time, he was near to tears. At this point, the doctor, who practised hypnosis, told Paul that it was possible to learn how to go into a nice dreamy state in which he would hardly be aware of what was going on. Would he like to do this? Yes, he would, he said. So Paul was asked to lie down on the couch and was put into hypnosis. Once he was in a trance, he was asked to imagine that he was sitting in front of the television at home, waiting for his favourite programme to come on. He was asked what the programme was and he said, 'Well, it's only just starting.'

'Can you see the titles coming up on the screen and hear the signature tune?'

'Yes.'

'Keep watching and listening, and as you do so the picture and the sound will become clearer and clearer until they will both be as clear as if you were watching the programme in front of your set at home. And you will find the programme so interesting and so enjoyable that you will not pay any attention to what I am doing. Even if you feel some discomfort, it won't worry you – you will be so interested in what's happening on the television that nothing will distract you from it until I tell you that it's time to wake up.'

And this is exactly what happened. Paul lay there, smiling to himself as he ran an edition of his favourite programme through his mind, and the doctor injected a local anaesthetic and incised and drained the abscess without the boy flinching once. When the wound had been dressed, Paul was told that the programme was finishing and that the closing credits were coming up. Then he was told to wake up and was asked how the programme had been and how he felt. 'Great!' was the answer to both questions.

This 'television' technique is one which is popular with dentists who treat children and is particularly useful when treatment is necessary which will entail the child either being in the chair for a long period of time or returning on several occasions. When a number of appointments are necessary, children may be asked to decide in advance which programme they want to watch on the next visit and, as a result, may almost look forward to their trips to the dentist.

Miss M. T.

Miss M. T. was a highly intelligent, well-educated young woman of 24 who worked as a translator for a large publishing house. While in her last year at university, she had met an American post-graduate student to whom she had been very attracted. They had gone out together on a regular basis during that year and, when he had returned to the United States, they had written to each other every two weeks or so. Four months before Miss M.T. went for hypnotherapy, her boyfriend had returned to England for an extended holiday during which he had proposed to her and she had accepted. Now he wanted her to go to America to meet his family, but she was terrified of flying. Her fiancé had already returned home and she would have to travel alone, which made the prospect even more alarming. Because she was under pressure at work, it was not possible for her to take more than a two-week break and so she could not go by boat. She would force herself to book her flight and get to the airport but she didn't know whether she could actually force herself to get on the plane – and if she couldn't, she would risk losing the man she loved.

Miss M. T. had flown twice before. At the age of fourteen she had taken a plane home from Paris where she had been on holiday with some relatives. They were staying in France for another week but she had to return to England for the start of the school term. On the outward journey they had travelled by car and boat but, since she would now be travelling alone, it was obviously easier for her to fly. She had not been nervous when she got on the plane but, unfortunately, the weather was bad and the flight was a very bumpy one. She sat next to a woman who regaled her with information about planes crashing in storms, and when she got off at the other end to be met by her parents, she was trembling and crying. After that she was able to avoid flying for seven years, but then had to fly to Edinburgh where her mother, who had been visiting a friend, had suddenly become seriously ill. On this occasion, Miss M. T. travelled with her father and, in view of her distress concerning her mother and her fear of flying, her GP had given her some tranquillizers to take for the journey. These had suppressed her panic to some extent but, when her mother had recovered, Miss M. T. was thankful to be able to return home on the train.

Her GP had suggested that she have some tranquillizers for her trip across the Atlantic but she was unwilling to take them on this occasion unless she absolutely had to. They had helped to control her anxiety when going to Edinburgh but she had felt very drowsy and 'like a zombie' on her arrival. Because the flight to the United States was so much longer than that to Edinburgh, she feared that she would have to take a larger dose of tranquillizers and that, by the time she arrived, she would be in no fit state to meet her future in-laws. It was then that her GP suggested that she might try some hypnotherapy.

When she went for her first session, she had managed to book her ticket and was intending to travel in three weeks' time. She had explained the delay to her fiancé by saying that she had some urgent work to complete before she could take any holiday. But if she delayed any longer, he would think that she was having second thoughts about marrying him.

Once in a hypnotic trance, Miss M. T. was told that in future she would not have any difficulty in relaxing and staying calm. (In fact, she was a very relaxed person and the only thing that made her panic was flying.) The sensation of relaxation and well-being was developed and then she was asked to visualize herself packing her suitcase, ready for her trip to the States. As she did so, suggestions were given to her that not only was she remaining relaxed, but she was getting quite excited at the thought of seeing her fiancé again and of meeting his family. Then the scene was shifted to the airport. She was told that it is natural, if we are under stress or having to do something out of the ordinary, for the body to release adrenaline into the system. When we are anxious or feel threatened, this can be an unpleasant sensation and can intensify the anxiety, but when we are happy, it can produce a feeling of excitement. In this case, because she was happy and looking forward to seeing her fiancé again, her mind would interpret the sensation as being one of excitement and it would add to her happiness. The visualization then continued along the lines described in the section on phobias in Chapter Six. Each time she started to feel nervous or apprehensive, she 'stopped' the scene until the sensation turned into one of excitement. Finally, she was able to picture herself getting onto the plane and starting the flight. She was asked to feel herself relax deeply and was able to report that she was feeling very calm and relaxed and comfortable. Then she was taught to hypnotize herself and was told that, once on the plane, she would be able to put herself into a trance and remain comfortably relaxed throughout the journey. She was told that she must tell the person sitting next to her what she was going to do and ask him to wake her up towards the end of the flight by touching her shoulder and saying, 'Wake up.' She could also ask him to do this when a meal was being served, so that she could wake up and eat. If she woke up to eat or if she needed to wake herself up to go to the toilet, she would remain quite calm all the time and would be able to go back into hypnosis as soon as she wanted to. Naturally, the therapist gave her the usual precautions concerning self-hypnosis, including, 'If anything should happen that needs your immediate attention, you will wake up immediately and, while remaining calm, will be fully alert to deal with it,' but of course he said it in such a way that it would not make her think that there was going to be an emergency on the plane! Finally, she was told that while she was in hypnosis the time would seem to go very quickly, although when she woke up it would return to its usual speed. Since she was a good subject, it seemed likely that she would be able to produce this time distortion.

Miss M. T. had two more sessions of hypnosis before her trip. On each occasion, the suggestions and techniques given at the first treatment were repeated. She practised her self-hypnosis diligently, and by the end of her third appointment she was feeling fairly confident about the trip.

When the time for her journey came, the flight was uneventful and she accomplished it with a minimum of anxiety. She was able to wake up for a meal but spent the rest of the time in hypnosis and found that it passed quickly.

She had a wonderful time in the States and coped well with the flight home. Three months later Miss M. T. and her fiancé were married – and flew to Bermuda for their honeymoon.

Mrs C. W.

Although hypnotherapy has its limitations, in that there are certain well-defined areas of illness in which it is not useful, the fact that it can be combined with other therapeutic techniques makes it very valuable in the treatment of a great variety of complaints. It can, of course, be used with many forms of orthodox medicine, but may also supplement other alternative therapies. Any therapy that uses visualization may be combined with hypnosis to very good effect. The use of visualization in the treatment of cancer, for example, was pioneered in the United States by Carl Simonton and Stephanie Matthews-Simonton (authors, with James L. Creighton, of *Getting Well Again*, Bantam, 1980) and their techniques would be quite suitable for use with hypnosis. Healing (called by various practitioners spiritual healing, psychic healing or hand healing) may also make use of visualizations through which the patient can use his own mind to help to heal his body.

Mrs C. W. was treated with a combination of hypnotherapy and a healing visualization. She went into her doctor's surgery one day with a nasty cut on her knee, having fallen over in the street. While the cut was being cleaned and stitched, she mentioned that she was 'always doing things like this'. She was, she said, very accident-prone. And many of the accidents were not, it seemed, of her own making. Hardly a day went by without something happening to her and she was getting heartily fed up with it. The day before she fell over in the street, someone had run into the back of her car when she had stopped at traffic lights. Two days before that, when changing the bed linen, one of the pillows had suddenly given way and filled the room with feathers. And to make matters worse, when she got out the vacuum cleaner to clear up the mess, she found that it wasn't working.

Now a healer might say that the reason that this lady was accident-prone was because she was surrounded by negative energies. The energy, or life force, that runs through the body has to flow in an ordered manner; if it is disrupted it can cause disease or abnormal mental states or, as in this case, can disturb the patient's environment. (The phenomenon of the poltergeist, when inanimate objects are hurled across the room and doors open and shut of their own accord, is often associated with the presence in the household of a disturbed teenager.) Mrs C. W.'s GP was a hypnotherapist with a knowledge of healing techniques. He felt that it would be appropriate to treat her with a healing visualization technique to allow her to realign her body energies, in conjunction with hypnosis, which would make the visualization easier for her to do and could also be used to give her ego-strengthening and to teach her to relax.

The method he used was based on a technique described in *The Psychic Healing Book* by Amy Wallace and Bill Henkin (Turnstone Press, 1981). Once Mrs C. W. was in hypnosis and had been given some basic suggestions concerning relaxation and for ego-strengthening, he asked her to focus on a point just in front of the base of her spine and, when she was aware of that point, to imagine that lying there was a cord which had been rolled up into a ball. He then asked her to run that cord out and to picture it running down through the chair on which she was sitting, into the ground and right down to the centre of the earth, where it would anchor itself. This cord could then be used for waste disposal, to get rid of all the disturbed energies which surrounded her. She was asked to imagine that she was sweeping round her body with her hands, scooping up any 'muck' that surrounded her and transferring it to the start of the cord. It would flow down the cord, just like rubbish going down a waste disposal unit, and when it got to the centre of the earth, it would disperse so that it could harm no one. When she had been all round her body with her imaginary hands, and had cleared away as much as she could, she was asked to draw up through her cord a clear, fresh, bubbling energy which she could use to wash through and round her body and which would flush any remaining garbage down the cord. She could repeat this step as many times as she needed to, flushing the used energy down the cord each time, until she felt clean and fresh. And then she was asked to draw up a final lot of energy which she could keep in her body. The doctor taught her to do self-hypnosis and suggested that each time she hypnotized herself she should use the cord technique to rid herself of any anxieties or tensions that she had picked up during the day.

Mrs C. W. was asked to return in two weeks and, when she did so, reported that she had had only one minor accident since her last appointment. She had been practising her self-hypnosis each day and was feeling confident that she had rid herself of her accident-prone tendency. She was told to continue to practise the technique and to return if the tendency showed any sign of coming back. However, she did not need another appointment. Six months later, she had to see her GP again as she had a bad cough, and she was able to report that she no longer seemed to be accident-prone.

Mrs S. H.

This 35-year-old lady was referred for hypnotherapy by her GP because she wanted to give up smoking. She had started to smoke when she was in her late teens, and although she had sometimes managed to give up for a few weeks she had always gone back to it. Her husband had died from leukaemia two years earlier after several months of illness, much of which was spent in hospital. About a year after his death, she had an attack of depression which quickly resolved itself when treated with a six-week course of antidepressant tablets. She worked as a buyer in a store and had two daughters aged 14 and 12.

Mrs S. H. was given the usual treatment for smokers, with suggestions on how easy it was going to be to give up, and was taught to hypnotize herself. Self-hypnosis can induce depression in susceptible patients, but in this case it seemed as though her one attack of depression had been a reaction to her husband's death and was unlikely to recur. However, as a precaution, when she had come out of the trance, she was warned that if she started to feel even the slightest bit depressed, she should stop her practice immediately.

Two weeks later she returned. Not only was she still smoking but she had become very depressed. When she had had the first attack of depression, she had accepted it as being 'one of those things', but its sudden recurrence after two sessions of self-hypnosis, together with what the therapist had told her, had made her start to wonder why she should be susceptible to depression, as it now appeared that she was. As a result, she had come to some surprising conclusions. She had not, she said, been very happy with her life since her husband had died, but she had become so used to bottling up her feelings that she was fooling even herself. She missed her husband more than she wanted to admit and therefore she had 'shut the emotions away'. She was asked whether she had really mourned her husband. No, she had shed a few tears, but all through his last illness she had tried to keep cheerful for him, and when he was gone she had tried to keep cheerful for the girls, who were quite distraught at losing their father. The therapist suggested that what she really needed was to allow herself to grieve. She agreed to talk to her daughters, who were sensible girls, about the fact that she sometimes felt very lonely and needed to cry. She was put into hypnosis and given suggestions that she would allow herself to weep and to mourn. But, by doing so, she would begin to feel great relief, as though a weight was lifting from her shoulders. Gradually all the sadness and pain would disappear and she would be left with happy memories of her husband. The grief at losing him would be replaced by a thankfulness that she had known him and loved him and been loved by him, and joy that he had given her two wonderful daughters.

Mrs S. H. was asked to get in touch again if she should need any further help but was not given another appointment. Six months later, a letter arrived in which she said that she had allowed herself to mourn and to grieve deeply, helped and supported by her daughters and by a close friend at work. She had now cast off the depression and could think of her husband with smiles rather than tears. She was a great deal happier than she had been for several years and, in the last three weeks, had given up smoking.

Mr N. B.

Mr N. B. requested hypnotherapy to help him stop smoking. He was a very good subject and it seemed as though he would have little difficulty in giving up, since he had the motivation to do so. At his second appointment, he mentioned that he was due to go into hospital as a day patient in order to have some little fatty nodules removed from under his eyes. He asked whether he might put himself into hypnosis for the duration of the operation, which was to be done under local anaesthetic. This seemed a very sensible idea: not only would he be very relaxed, but hypnosis also has the effect of controlling bleeding, and this might help to reduce the bruising that was likely to occur afterwards. (The area around the eyes is very sensitive and Mr N. B. had been warned that he might have considerable bruising for a week or so after the operation.) When he arrived at the hospital for his operation, he spoke to the surgeon and, finding that he had no objection, put himself into a trance while the fatty lumps were removed.

A week later he returned for another session of hypnotherapy, by which time he had stopped smoking. The therapist asked about the operation and was told that all had gone very well. Not only had he remained perfectly relaxed and comfortable during the operation, but, somewhat to the surgeon's surprise, he had developed no bruising whatsoever.

CHAPTER EIGHT

HOW TO FIND

A THERAPIST

AND WHAT

TO EXPECT

It is only in the last 20 years that hypnotherapy has started to become 'respectable'. Many doctors and psychotherapists all over the world are discovering its value and either using it themselves or referring patients to hypnotherapists. Even so, there are still doubts. I know of one patient who was referred by his G P to another doctor who practised acupuncture. The patient discovered that this doctor also practised hypnotherapy and when, some time later, he decided that he wanted to give up smoking, asked his G P to refer him back. The request was refused: the G P was quite happy to refer patients for acupuncture but not for hypnotherapy, which, he said, was a form of 'quackery' – even though, in this case, both were practised by the same respectable medical practitioner!

However, in some respects hypnotherapy has more in common with orthodox medicine than with other alternative therapies. In such therapies as homoeopathy, acupuncture and healing, the aim of treatment is to return the patient to as near normal a state as possible. But in orthodox medicine, although some forms of treatment may cure the patient, some may only control the condition (for example in high blood pressure or arthritis) and some may just alleviate the symptoms. Similarly, in some cases it may be possible for hypnosis to effect a cure (as in the treatment of phobias or chronic anxiety, where the patient can be helped to recognize and conquer the cause), but some conditions may only be controlled (for example migraine or asthma, where the patient may need to use a certain technique every time an attack begins in order to stop it from developing). And in some cases hypnosis will only alleviate the symptoms – as in the treatment of chronic pain.

However, like orthodox medicine, hypnotherapy can be useful in all three situations. Where the patient has tried every other available treatment without success, even a therapy that only controls the condition or alleviates the symptoms will be welcome. So when should one consider having hypnotherapy and when should one try another alternative therapy? Should hypnosis always be a last resort? The answer to this second question is definitely no. Any patient whose condition is directly related to stress or anxiety might be well advised to try hypnotherapy first. For a patient who suffers from a physical condition such as asthma, which is aggravated by anxiety or stress, hypnosis can be very successfully combined with orthodox treatment.

In the treatment of pain, hypnotherapy should probably come last on the list, simply because all it will do is cover up the symptoms. However, even here there may be cases, such as that of the woman who suffered from back pain (described in Chapter Seven), in which anxiety and tension play such a large part in the production of the pain that hypnotherapy may relieve it simply by teaching the patient how to relax. Normally, for back problems, osteopathy or chiropractic would probably be the treatment of first choice, but in this case her severe muscle spasm prevented the patient from responding.

The cases in which hypnotherapy excels are those in which the patient is suffering from anxiety and does not wish to take tranquillizers. Nowadays many doctors are becoming increasingly reluctant to prescribe tranquillizers and are happy to refer patients for other, non-addictive, forms of treatment.

It is possible nowadays to buy self-hypnosis tapes in shops and by mail order. Some people who have tried these and found them unhelpful may ask whether they are likely to fare any better with hypnotherapy. The answer to this is that although these tapes, which are now becoming increasingly popular, may be very helpful for some people, their use is limited. They may, certainly, induce a light hypnotic trance, and some patients who simply need to relax or who are trying to give up smoking may find that they are perfectly adequate for their purposes. However, most patients who have had hypnotherapy will say that the trances that they induce themselves are never as deep as those induced by the therapist. It does seem that better results are to be achieved from a session with a therapist than from a session, or sessions, with a tape recorder. In addition, the session that you have with a hypnotherapist is tailor-made for your own personal problems. In the case of a smoker, mention will be made of the times at which he finds it most difficult to refrain from smoking and specific suggestions can be given to help him to deal with them. If the patient is suffering from a particular mental or physical condition, specific suggestions appropriate to his own case are even more important. If a patient suspects that he is depressed, he should not try a self-hypnosis tape, and if he starts to feel depressed after using one, he should stop using it immediately. However, in the majority of cases, these tapes are harmless and may be helpful.

Having decided that one might benefit from hypnotherapy, how easy is it to find a therapist? Should one look in the small ads of the local paper, or in the Yellow Pages? As a general rule of thumb, most practitioners of alternative therapies, if they have been properly trained and registered, are not allowed to advertise. The Yellow Pages doesn't count as advertising so qualified therapists may appear there, but it may be difficult to distinguish them from any others. If one simply wants help to give up smoking, then probably the worst that can happen if one goes to an un-qualified or inadequately trained practitioner is that the therapy won't work. However, if one needs treatment for a medical condition or an anxiety state or phobia, it is very important to find a practitioner who has had the training appropriate to the treatment. In such cases, it is probably best to go to a doctor or psychotherapist. Psychiatry forms an important part of every doctor's training and many, especially if they intend to become GPs, spend six months working on a psychiatric ward after they have qualified. In addition, of course, they are able to assess a patient's physi-cal condition and the extent to which it is being affected by his mental state.

To be seen by a medical hypnotherapist you need a re-ferral from your own doctor, who may know of someone working in your area to whom he can send you. If a GP does not know any hypnotherapists, he can contact the British Society of Medical and Dental Hypnosis which keeps a list of doctors and dentists who practise the therapy. Some patients may prefer to go to a non-medical therapist, particularly if they require treatment for something simple (such as smoking) or if a particular therapist has been re-commended by a friend. However, not all these therapists have been trained to the same standard. There are many colleges of hypnotherapy in Britain, offering courses of differing lengths. Some teach only the theory and do not supervise the student's practical work. The fairly recently formed Association of Professional Therapists is hoping to compile a national register of hypnotherapists who have qualified from an accredited training scheme or have had many years of experience; in order to appear on the register, a therapist will also have to work in suitable premises and observe a strict code of conduct. Members of the British Hypnotherapy Association, who use the letters MBHA after their names, are trained psychotherapists. The addresses of these organizations appear at the end of the book.

Many dentists are using hypnosis nowadays to treat dental phobias and to relieve pain during dental treatment. The British Society of Medical and Dental Hypnosis can supply the names and addresses of these dentists. Since you can change your dentist at will, no letter of referral is required. Officially, no dentist is allowed to treat conditions that come outside his scope. However, some may help patients to give up smoking, although they will not tackle more psychotherapeutic or medical treatments. Occasionally a dentist may find that an initial interest in hypnotherapy leads him into other fields, so that it may be possible to find a dentist who is also a trained psychotherapist and treats all manner of conditions.

The cost of hypnotherapy will vary from therapist to therapist. Many practitioners offer reduced rates to patients who cannot afford the full fees, and patients to whom this applies should always enquire about it when they make their first appointment. The session itself also varies according to the individual therapist and, of course, the condition that he happens to be treating. However, as a general rule, one can say that the first session will last about an hour and, being longer than subsequent sessions, will be more expensive. On this occasion the therapist will take a very full history from the patient and may enquire into his family background and childhood as well as noting the details of the present problem. Some practitioners do not give any treatment at the first session but simply explain to patients the lines upon which they intend to treat them. A young child may be given the option of delaying treatment until the second session, and this is often helpful in building up his confidence in the practitioner. If treatment is given at the first session, it is usually quite short since there is often little time left once the history has been taken. The patient will be put into hypnosis, perhaps given a few suggestions concerning relaxation, and may be taught to hypnotize himself.

It is on the second visit that the work usually begins. From this session on, the patient may expect to be seen for about half an hour, most of which will be taken up by treatment. The treatment itself will, of course, depend on the condition being treated, but many therapists teach self-hypnosis and give the patient suggestions that he can repeat to himself while he is doing his practice. Some practitioners like to make a cassette recording of the hypnotherapy session so that the patient can play it back at home and thus have a 'self-hypnosis' session which is identical to that which he has with the therapist.

The length of treatment and frequency of sessions depend very much on the individual patient and his complaint. Patients are often seen at weekly or fortnightly intervals to begin with and then, as their condition starts to improve, less often. Some patients may need to continue treatment for many months, particularly those who are suffering from severe and chronic phobias. Others, such as those who wish to give up smoking, may need only two or three sessions. Whatever the condition being treated, one would normally expect some improvement, even if only very slight, within four or five sessions. No change in the condition after five sessions suggests that perhaps the patient should be trying a different therapy. There are, of course, some conditions that hypnosis cannot help and may make worse. The most important of these is depression; schizophrenia is another. This is why it may be inadvisable to see a hypnotherapist without speaking to your doctor first.

It is important to remember that hypnotherapy is not a cure-all and has definite limitations. However, alone or combined with other therapies, it may produce a dramatic improvement in a patient's condition, especially when that condition is aggravated by stress.

USEFUL ADDRESSES

Registers of Practitioners

Medical and dental hypnotherapists

British Society of Medical and Dental Hypnosis, PO Box 6, 42 Links Road, Ashtead, Surrey KT21 2HT

Psychotherapists

National Council of Psychotherapists and Hypnotherapy Register, The Glebe House, Pevensey, Sussex (Eastbourne 762360)

Lay hypnotherapists

Association of Professional Therapists, 37B New Cavendish Street, London, W1M 8JR

Training Organizations

For doctors and dentists

British Society of Medical and Dental Hypnosis (address above)

For psychotherapists and psychoanalysts

British Hypnotherapy Association, 67 Upper Berkeley Street, London W1 (01-723 4443)

Index

Adrenaline, 53–5
Agoraphobia, 130
Allergens, experiments with, 57–8
Analgesia, 133
Animal magnetism, 19
Anxiety, 107–11, 135
Asthma, 47, 55, 111–15, 147–51
Aura, 63
Autonomic nervous system, 51–6

Bedwetting, see Enuresis
Berlin Academy of Sciences, 23
Bernheim, Hippolyte-Marie, 39
Bloxham, Arnall, 89, 95
Bonding, 114–15, 148–50
Braid, James, 37–8
Brain, left and right sides, 60
Bramwell, James Milne, 42–3
Breuer, Joseph, 40–41
British Association for the Advancement of Science, 38
British Dental Association, 44
British Dental Journal, 43
British Medical Association, 41–2, 44
British Medical Journal, 42
British Society of Dental Hypnosis, 43, 44, 45
British Society of Medical and Dental Hypnosis, 45, 79–80
Buddhist meditation, 63

Catharsis, 41
Central nervous system, 49–50
Charcot, Jean Martin, 39–40, 41
Chastenet de Puysegur, Marquis, 30

Deepening techniques, 67–70
De la suggestion, 39
D'Eslon, Charles, 26, 27–8
Di Faria, Abbé José Custodio, 29–30
Duodenal (peptic) ulcer, 47, 55
Dupotet de Sennevoy, Baron, 30

Eczema, 118–19
Ego-strengthening, 70–72
Electro-encephalogram: in hypnosis, 59, 64; in meditation, 64
Elliotson, John, 30–34
Enuresis, 120–23
Esdaile, James, 34–7

Faculty of Medicine, French, 27, 28
Federation of Stage Hypnotists, 79–80
Fiore, Edith, 87–8, 93
Forel, Auguste, 40
Freud, Sigmund, 41

Gall, Franz Joseph, 31

Hallucinations, 118–19, 126–7
Hand levitation, 69–70
Harveian Oration, 33
Hell, Father Maximilian, 20
Holism, 48–9
Hypnosis: for children, 112, 118; definition of, 56–7; and dentistry, 43, 44, 133, 155; effect on memory, 81–4; forensic, 82–3; group therapy in, 112; and healing, 23–4; and meditation, 63–4; in obstetrics, 131–2; operations under, 33, 35–6, 153–5, 163–4
Hypnosis in Medicine and Surgery, see *Mesmerism in India*
Hypnotherapy session, 66, 75
Hypnotic suggestion, 16–18
Hypnotic trance, 15–16; depth of, 18, 65–6; memory of; 18–19; waking up from, 14–15
Hypnotism Act (1952), 75
Hysteria, 40

Ichthyosiform erythrodermia of Brocq, 119–20

FOR THE BEST IN PAPERBACKS, LOOK FOR THE 🐧

In every corner of the world, on every subject under the sun, Penguin represents quality and variety – the very best in publishing today.

For complete information about books available from Penguin – including Pelicans, Puffins, Peregrines and Penguin Classics – and how to order them, write to us at the appropriate address below. Please note that for copyright reasons the selection of books varies from country to country.

In the United Kingdom: For a complete list of books available from Penguin in the U.K., please write to *Dept E.P., Penguin Books Ltd, Harmondsworth, Middlesex, UB7 0DA*

In the United States: For a complete list of books available from Penguin in the U.S., please write to *Dept BA, Penguin, 299 Murray Hill Parkway, East Rutherford, New Jersey 07073*

In Canada: For a complete list of books available from Penguin in Canada, please write to *Penguin Books Canada Ltd, 2801 John Street, Markham, Ontario L3R 1B4*

In Australia: For a complete list of books available from Penguin in Australia, please write to the *Marketing Department, Penguin Books Australia Ltd, P.O. Box 257, Ringwood, Victoria 3134*

In New Zealand: For a complete list of books available from Penguin in New Zealand, please write to the *Marketing Department, Penguin Books (NZ) Ltd, Private Bag, Takapuna, Auckland 9*

In India: For a complete list of books available from Penguin, please write to *Penguin Overseas Ltd, 706 Eros Apartments, 56 Nehru Place, New Delhi, 110019*

In Holland: For a complete list of books available from Penguin in Holland, please write to *Penguin Books Nederland B.V., Postbus 195, NL–1380AD Weesp, Netherlands*

In Germany: For a complete list of books available from Penguin, please write to *Penguin Books Ltd, Friedrichstrasse 10 – 12, D–6000 Frankfurt Main 1, Federal Republic of Germany*

In Spain: For a complete list of books available from Penguin in Spain, please write to *Longman Penguin España, Calle San Nicolas 15, E–28013 Madrid, Spain*